MW00737082

FACIAL REFLEXOLOGY

Lone Sorensen

World's First Facial Reflexologist

Third Edition

HEALTH 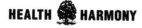 HARMONY

An imprint of

B. Jain Publishers (P) Ltd.

USA — EUROPE — INDIA

FACIAL REFLEXOLOGY

Lone Sorensen
Facial Reflexology sorensensistemTM: A book about facial therapy.
Copyright 2002 Lone Sorensen

First Edition: 2008
Second Edition: 2009
Third Edition: 2011
3rd Impression: 2014

Information:
Lone Sorensen
Sorensensistem
Lope de Vega 6
08005 Barcelona
Spain

Tel: (0034) 933078972, (0034) 678769550
E-mail: sorensensistem@post.tele.dk
www.reflexologiafacial.es/www.facialreflexologyusa.com
www.lonesorensen.com/www.globalfacial.com

Models:
Melisa Liberti
Estefania Vaucheret

Illustrations and Photography:
Christian Johnsen

Design:
Sebastian Jimenez
Vijesh Chahal

Published by Kuldeep Jain for :

HEALTH HARMONY

An imprint of
B. JAIN PUBLISHERS (P) LTD.
1921/10, Chuna Mandi, Paharganj, New Delhi 110 055 (INDIA)
Tel.: 91-11-4567 1000
Fax: 91-11-45671010 • *E-mail:* info@bjain.com
Website: **www.bjain.com**

Printed in India by:
J.J. Offset Printers

ISBN: 978-81-319-1167-9

Publisher's Note

As the civilization moves into the next century, it is evident that the role of medical and health care system is also changing drastically.

The medical system has grown manifolds with improvement in technology which has lead to an increase in the average life span. However, inspite of improvements in technology, the number of diseases and their complexities are still on a rise. Modern medicine has provided answers to many such conditions but many diseases still remain uncured. Here comes the role of therapies beyond modern medicine.

Facial Reflexology is one such therapy which works efficiently for the treatment of various diseases and can be given in conjugation with conventional medicine.

Lone Sorensen is a trained reflexologist. She has been a key person in establishing first three reflexology schools and has trained over two thousand students over a period of twelve years.

She is first reflexologist to be awarded with three Honorary titles by OMHS (A Humanitarian and Health Organization).

We are glad to be the publishers for her work which we hope will be a step towards better health for humanity.

Kuldeep Jain
C.E.O., B. Jain Publishers (P) Ltd.

Acknowledgement

My Thanks to

Maria Snaiderman, reflexologist and assistant, Argentina.

Pilar Rios, reflexologist and assistant, Argentina.

Fabian Pico, doctor and assistant, Argentina.

Carlos Chesñevar, The University of Rector, Argentina.

Dr Philip, Pinel Foundation, Bs. As., Argentina.

Carla Rodiguez, graphic designer, Argentina.

Christian Johnsen, photos and graphics, Spain.

Also to

Zandra Willumsen, reflexology teacher, Denmark.

Sport Lesions Clinic, Dorthe Kirkebaekke, Denmark.

Henning Mørkeberg, therapist, Denmark.

For their support.

Foreword

In my twenty years of profession as a reflexologist and the owner of the Danish School of Zone therapy in Copenhagen, I have never met an able therapist and teacher as enthusiastic as Lone Sorensen. With Facial Reflexology therapy, her book and her courses, she has created a new world for therapists and a fantastic tool as a gift for humanity. Not to mention, she has helped many children and adults with different handicaps with Facial Reflexology across the world. The book is an insight into the ancient Indian treating technique co-ordinated with oriental medicine, which gives us deeper insight to the healing process inside human body.

Prof. Zandra Willumsen
Den Danske Zoneterapeut Skole Aps

Preface

This book aims to introduce **Facial Reflexology**, also known as **Facial Therapy**, to explain the technique and to trace its beginnings. With over twenty eight years of intensive work, it has evolved into a professional and effective therapy. Curiosity, research and a lot of clinical experience has led me to combine ancient methods (from all over the world) with modern techniques. I do not pretend to present a detailed account of neurology, acupuncture or zone therapy, my intention is to give a detailed summary of the various techniques of facial reflexology. The results obtained with facial reflexology are of organic, physical, chemical and neurological nature. Facial reflexology has also proved to be very effective in the rehabilitation of patients with brain injuries and neurological problems.

My work and my methods have been recognized at an international level. In March 2001, I was awarded three honorary titles by a Humanitarian and Health Organization (OMHS) in Argentina, making me the first reflexologist to be awarded. Facial Reflexology was introduced in Latin America and Europe in 1996, at various national conferences for children with disabilities.

The content of this book is based on my clinical experiences gained over the last many years. From 1979 to 1988, I worked principally with children suffering from learning and behavior difficulties in Denmark. I then spent 12 years in Argentina as the first reflexologist in the country where I treated patients with brain damage and neurological problems. Over this period, I opened three schools and trained two thousand reflexologists.

I then spent two years working on projects at the Kurhuset Rehabilitation Centre in Philadelphia, Denmark and at my clinic in Copenhagen teaching my technique mainly to parents of children with brain damage and trained therapists, something that I still carry out in my school in Barcelona, and also at The Medical Faculty at the University Complutense in Madrid.

I studied reflexology, acupuncture and kinesiology in Denmark and perfected my knowledge of oriental medicine, facial acupuncture, auricular acupuncture, vibrational therapy, neurology and anatomy in places as far apart as Cuba, France, Spain, Germany and Argentina.

This book is a compendium based on my practical experiences, theories, research and studies carried out since 1978. It does not teach the rehabilitation techniques for patients with brain damage but shows the basic technique that can be used to deal with various types of problems. It is based on more than one hundred thousand treatments carried out on people, and supervised by myself.

My aim is to make the masses aware about this treatment that has over the years helped so many people, adults and children alike. I have been fortunate enough to have at my disposal many patients who offered selflessly and trustingly their feet, hands and faces so that I could research the points and nerves, with the precise intention of seeing the interconnections between the oriental, Indian and today´s neurological methods.

I am thankful to my assistants in Argentina for the knowledge I possess today.

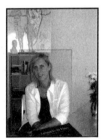

Lone Sorensen
Sorensensistem
Lope de Vega 6
08005 Barcelona
Spain

Facial Reflexology

Facial reflexology is a therapeutic method in which stimulation of zones and points of the face are utilized to alleviate health conditions in other parts of the body. Originally, it is based upon the ancient Chinese, Vietnamese and Aboriginal practice. The somatopic correspondence of specific parts of the body to specific parts of the face was first developed in the Oriental medicine. It is this integrated system of oriental and western practices of facial therapy, which will be described in the text that follows.

Complementary Medical Modalities Used With Facial Reflexology

Acupuncture
Chiropractic
Nursing
Reflexology
Dentistry
Naturopathy
Orthopedics
Physiotherapy
Psychotherapy

Contents

CHAPTER 1

Introduction to Facial Reflexology

Reflexology is the practice of manual therapies in various forms and their application on different parts of body including face, hands and feet, dates back to over 3,000 years, ago primarily in the studies of Egyptian, African and Aboriginal cultures as well as their mythologies.

The oldest documentation describing the practice of reflexology takes us to Egypt. A drawing dated around 2500 BC, found in the tomb of a distinguished Egyptian Doctor, **Anknahor de Saqqara** shows the practice of foot and facial reflexology in his surgery.

In some parts of South America, which were occupied by the **Incas**, reflexology was used as a preventative health treatment through generations. For hundreds of years, the **Cherokee Indians** in Carolina, North America, recognized the importance of maintaining a physical, mental and spiritual balance. As a means to this end, they practised reflexology. The **Oso clan**, descendants of the *Cherokees* (who nowadays inhabit the hills of Allehjanies) practised *'zone therapy'* on the feet. Infact, the most well known therapist of zone therapy working today in America is Jenny Wallace, a Cherokee Indian. There are other aboriginal cultures in the Andes, southern Argentina who still use facial therapy in its primitive form.

It was not until 1800 that reflexology was introduced into Europe. The first medical practitioner to use facial reflexology in

Europe was a German Doctor, **Dr Alfonso Cornelius**. He suffered a serious infection and cured himself by stimulating different points and areas of his face. He went on to practise the treatment with significant results. Infact he was the first person in Europe to publish an article on facial reflex therapy. The article, entitled '**Druckpunte**', was published in 1902 in a monthly medical magazine.

In 1872, an American doctor, **William Fitzgerald**, educated at the University of Medicine in Vermont, was conducting research into reflexology in Vienna and London and he came up with some interesting results especially with regards to ear, nose and throat.

In the 20th Century, two American doctors, **George Goodhart** and **John F. Thei** carried out a research on acupuncture and created a technique known as *'Kinesiology'*, which includes the stimulation of the cranium. *'Cranial sacral therapy'*, was also developed in the 20th Century, which occupies an important place amongst complementary medicine in the world today.

To understand reflex therapy, one has to go back over 5,000 years in history. It was created and developed over several hundred years in oriental villages. Manual reflex therapy was created long time before acupuncture. In fact, it is the oldest form of traditional oriental medicine. There are references even during Stone Age, regarding the use of sharp stones, thorns and other instruments to alleviate pain and diseases. There are also ancient references illustrating ways of diagnosing a patient by observing their ear, tongue and face, and by feeling the pulses at different points of the body. Modern facial reflexology is an amalgamation of the methods used by the South American Indians, Egyptians and the Orientals, together with the latest concepts of neuroanatomy.

The most important oriental techniques of reflexology are acupuncture, cranial acupressure, cerebral acupuncture, facial acupuncture and nasal therapy.

MICRO-SYSTEM THEORY OF FACE REFLEXOLOGY

Not only the face, but every part of the gross anatomy can function as an energetic system for diagnosis and therapy. This system is called micro-puncture and is different from the traditional Chinese system which is called a macro-system, where invisible lines or meridians cross the body. The meridians connect acupuncture points distributed throughout the body. The micro-systems have holographic distribution of points and the topography of points reiterates the anatomy of the body. The micro-puncture systems have been identified on the ear, foot, hand, face, nose, abdomen, back, iris, tongue, wrist, teeth, scalp, neck, temporal bone, lips and on every long and short bone of the body.

Every micro-system manifests neurological reflexes that are connected with the parts of the body. These reflexes are diagnostic and therapeutic and may be stimulated by finger pressure, needle acupuncture, heat, electrical stimulation, laser stimulation, magnets, or any method utilized by *macro-acupuncture*.

The micro-system is a reflex map of the body and replicates the anatomical arrangement of the whole body. '*Soma*' refers to the body, and '*Topography*' refers to mapping the terrain of an area. Micro-systems are connected to the Somatotopic neurological reflexes in the brain, where a picture of a homunculus or a map of a little man can be identified by brain mapping studies.

The micro-systems have bilateral effects, but they are usually more reactive when the micro-acupoint and the area of body pathology are ipsilateral to each other. The scalp micro-system, which corresponds to the underlying cerebral cortex is the principal system in which the side of the micro-system reflex is contralateral to the side of body.

All micro-systems function like echo resonators from the skin to the corresponding body organs, comparable to the echo resonance of wave form interference patterns in a hologram. Health problems in a specific organ or part of the body are indicated by distinct changes in the skin at the corresponding micro-system points, in an organ-cutaneous reflex. These localized skin changes may include increased tenderness on palpitation, altered blood flow, elevated temperature, changes in ectodermal activity, or changes in skin color or texture. Localized skin changes are diagnostically useful for all micro-systems. This stimulation triggers connections from nervous system to the spinal cord and brain, which in turn activates bio-energetic transformations, biochemical releases and electrical firing of neuronal reflexes. The organic reflex initiates pain relief and healing effects in the same ways as the macro-systems function.

All the micro-systems are interactive with the macro-systems. Treatment of one system will produce changes in the body's energetic patterns as diagnosed by the other systems. Facial Reflexology is the micro-system formed by other different micro-systems and in the following pages, you will find an introduction of the systems used to form the new and modern Facial Reflexology.

Cranial Acupunture and Acupressure

Cerebral acupuncture and cranial acupressure are techniques recently expounded by Chinese doctors. The neurologist, **Chia Shun Fa**, working from a hospital in the district of Ji, in Shan Xi, successfully treated individuals with brain injuries using acupuncture techniques.

In 1973, The Institute of Traditional Chinese Medicine in Shanghai published its first paper about Cranial Acupressure. In the same year, the first research to take place in the West on cranial acupressure was being done by a **Dr Claude Roustand** during the first Congress of the USMA in Monaco. Dr Roustand and Dr Nguyen Van Nghy were the doctors responsible for introducing the techniques to the West.

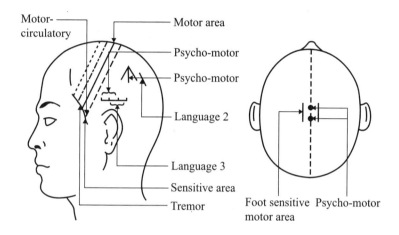

Illustration: Cranial acupressure and cerebral acupuncture, Dr Chia Shun Fa. 1973, Institute of Traditional Medicine

Cranial acupressure is based on studies of the relationship between the cerebral cortex and the scalp. The treatment is localized on the cranium, the surface of the skin and the structures of the cerebral cortex.

Scalp acupuncture has been particularly effective in treating strokes and cerebrovascular conditions. While there are two scalp micro-systems, the principal system divides the temporal section of the scalp in three parts. A diagonal line is extended laterally from the top of the head to the area of the temples above the ear. The lowest portion of this temporal line relates to the head, the middle area relates to the body, arms and hands, and the uppermost region represents the legs and feet, which is thus in an inverted body orientation. This Scalp system connects reflexes in the somatotropic cerebral cortex to the contra-lateral side of the body.

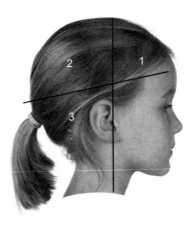

Illustration: *The principal system dividing the scalp into three parts*

Nasal Therapy

The first description of nasal therapy appeared in China in the texts of **Neijing Suwen** and **Neijing Lingshu**, where they explained the evidence of a double system of protection for the nose and face. The treatment consists of simply stimulating twenty four different zones of the face, nose and surrounding area.

Nasal therapy is also practised in India and Egypt, and is related to reflexology and the techniques of acupuncture and moxibustion. The method works on the specific area being touched, and at the same time has an effect on other parts and systems of the body such as the respiratory, cardiovascular, digestive, gynecological, nervous system etc. Amongst the big names practising nasal therapy in the 20th Century are two French doctors – **Dr Paul Gillet** and **Dr Vidal**.

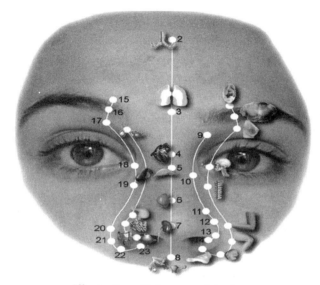

Illustration: *Hologram of the face*

Face and Nose Systems from Chinese researchers have identified micro-systems on the face and nose that are oriented in an upright position. The hologram of the face system places the head and neck in the forehead, the lungs between the eyebrows, the heart on the bridge of the nose, and the urogenital system in the philtrum (between the lips and nose). In the hologram of the nose system; the midline points are the same as in the face system, the digestive system is at the wings of the nose, and the upper and lower extremities are in the crease along the sides of the nose.

Facial Acupuncture

The oldest Facial acupuncture we know consists about twenty four points divided into four areas on the face:

The *nasal front area*, which in nasal therapy corresponds to the forehead (7 points). The *Ocular area,* with 8 points and the *Labial area*, which encircles some of the points on the lateral line of the wing of the nose (4 points). The *Chin area*, corresponds to the zygomatic apophysis (5 points). To facilitate the finding of the points, the face can be divided into a grid. The illustration below shows the first map made by **Dr Zhen Jui Xui** in 1974, at the Institute of Chinese Medicine in Shanghai.

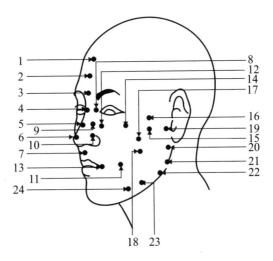

1.	Cranium	13.	Hips
2.	Tonsils	14.	Colon
3.	Lungs	15.	Feet
4.	Sinuses	16.	Kidneys
5.	Liver	17.	Arms
6.	Gall bladder	18.	Hands
7.	Spleen	19.	Palms of the hands
8.	Stomach	20.	Navel
9.	Bladder/a	21.	Muscles
10.	Bladder/b	22.	Knees
11.	Small intestine	23.	Knee joints
12.	Shoulders	24.	Legs

Illustration: Dr Zhen Jui Xue's twenty four facial points

Auricular Acupuncture

Auricular acupuncture is a two thousand year old therapy associated with traditional Chinese medicine. However, the techniques were modernized in 1950's. Nowadays, doctors and researchers in Shangtung use the technique with notable success.

In France, **Dr Nogier** developed his method of auricular medicine and thus, two methods of auricular acupuncture exist today. It is the most well known and used technique within the so called 'micro-systems' and is a therapy which is frequently used in combination with facial reflexology.

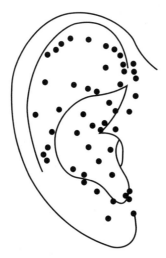

Illustration: *Auricular acupuncture points*

The Indian Zone Therapy

An important component of facial reflexology involves applying a technique, which was practised by aboriginal Indians in South America. The method is not only based on the manual stimulation of different areas of the face with the aim of regulating the functioning of the body at an organic, physical, chemical and psychological level but it is also used as an important tool of diagnosis. In the modern method of Facial Reflexology, this technique is used as the second step. The names of the seventeen different facial zones explain the connections via the central nervous system to all the systems of the body.

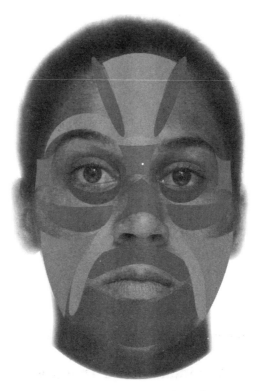

Illustration: *The first map showing the Indian zone therapy*

CHAPTER 2

First Step to Facial Reflexology

My idea for facial reflexology began in 1978. I had recently completed my training as a foot reflexologist in Copenhagen, Denmark, and had gone on to study acupuncture, kinesiology, craniosacral therapy and laser therapy. Later, I opened my own clinic and employed experienced therapists to work along side with me. We treated children with deportment behaviour and learning difficulties and it was during this time that I developed my first map of the face. I spent ten years studying and working in my native country, where I learnt a lot by combining foot reflexology with the points on the face, something that proved helpful in my later research.

In 1988 I moved to Bahia Blanca in Argentina, where I opened a clinic, unaware of the fact that reflexology was a completely unknown therapy there. These with the success that I had in treating patients, word soon spread and with that came more patients, which gave me an opportunity to develop the system professionally. The type of problems I encountered were very different from the health problems of my patients in Denmark. In Argentina, I had the opportunity of treating people with very grave and complicated illnesses, patients with brain damage and with terminal illnesses. This drove me to study and to research extensively into neurology and the techniques used in oriental medicine.

The same year, I travelled to the south with the intention of visiting the volcanic hot springs in Cophau de los Andes. They are the only one of their kind in the world and are known for their curative properties. This fascinating and beautiful place is two thousand metres above sea level in the middle of the mountains. Eleven volcanic hot springs, each with distinct properties, colours and temperatures along with steam, the smell of sulphur and the sound of boiling water, gave the place a special ambience.

In ancient times, the hot springs were used by the Indians for generations. People who continue to live in the south of the Andes as nomads, live in tents and move each month further north, according to the changes in temperature and the snow. They live on fish caught from rivers and make tents and clothes from lamb's wool and leather.

During my first visit to the hot springs, I managed to get close to a group of Indians who were camped very near to the centre of the springs. With great surprise, I watched some of the women treating each other with facial therapy. Sitting on the ground with their legs crossed, bearing the head of another Indian women in her lap. I watched as they worked, passing their hands over the faces in an orderly way and with movements that I had never seen before. I could guess fromthe way she looked at me that I was welcome.

Later, I often visited their camp with a pen and paper in hand, always at the same hour to observe. Each time the woman would be working on a different person. The other Indians in the camp looked at me with the same interest as I looked at them, all the time making me feel that I was welcome.

For two years I continued to visit them, trying to learn their technique and later trying it in combination with my map of facial points, on my patients in Bahia Blanca. The results were impressive, particularly with patients suffering from brain damage and neurological disorders.

In 1991, I travelled to Cuba to learn about their rehabilitation techniques. Working daily with the same patients suffering from injury, I made some fantastic observations. There were two reasons for their success; *firstly*, the amount of time they spent treating each patient was up to eight hours per day and *secondly*, their acupuncture and reflex therapy techniques were of a very high standard.

During this visit I learned **Dr Bui Quoc Chau's** method of facial acupunture, facial zone therapy and a neurological facial map with its 564 points, something which proved very important in my development of facial reflexology.

Dr Chau was a Vietnamese doctor, practicing in a hospital in Saigon in the 1980's. Dr Chau, with, his team of doctors developed a method called *'Cibernetic'*. The technique includes elements of acupuncture, western medicine, neurology and reflexology. While studying the relationship between the face and the body, Dr Chau identified more than five hundred points on the face. The points on the map are directly related to the central nervous system and the cerebral cortex, thus explaining the reason why the results are so quick and effective. Touching the points on the face, sends information immediately to the organs and systems of the body.

The method Cibernetics, includes stimulating the different areas and also incorporates a diagnostic technique. It is a complicated method which requires years of studying acupuncture and medicine. However, a part of the Cibernetic technique, known as *Cibertherapy*, is available without too extensive study of medicine and furthermore is compatible with other therapies. The treatment includes autostimulation, using either needles, fingertips, laser or electroacupressure, to further encourage the stimulation.

The Vietnamese maps of the zones on the face match Meridianology and central nervous system, both comprising the basic techniques of facial reflexology. I cross checked the neurological points on the map of 564 points with the symptoms and pathology of the patient.

In Cuba, they have been using acupuncture and reflexology techniques in the rehabilitation of patients since 1962 with excellent results. It was **Dr Florea Caballo**, who was responsible for obtaining recognition of acupuncture in Cuba. In 1993, I travelled again to Cuba and took part in an interesting course on the Ryodotten method of stimulation and diagnosis developed by **Dr Yoshio Nakatanis**.

'Ryodotten' means stimulation through hyper electric conductors. I had personally been working with electro-stimulation and laser therapy since 1984, and Dr Yoshio's ideas confirmed my own experiences on the importance of electro-stimulation.

During these years, I formed a new map of neurological points on the feet and hands based on the observations and results that I got from using this type of therapy. Combined with facial reflexology and other reflex therapies, they jointly form the basic treatment nowadays that are used in the rehabilitation of patients suffering from brain damage, whether it is damage as a result of an accident or from birth, a therapy known as **'Temprana therapy'** is used.

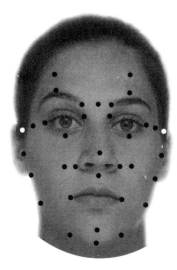

Illustration: *NP points used in the basic stimulation of facial reflexology. They are called neurovascular points because they access two systems – neurological and vascular system*

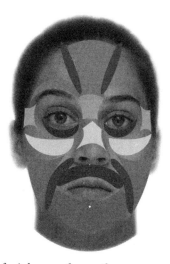

Illustration: *A facial map of zone therapy, as used in the South American Indian culture. The location of the zones is based upon the positioning of the organs in the body*

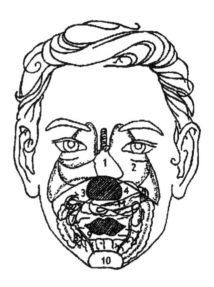

Illustration: The original Vietnamese map: The areas correspond to the main meridians/vital organs

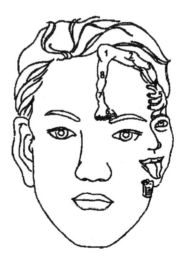

Illustration: The original Vietnamese map of the cortex and the cranial nerves

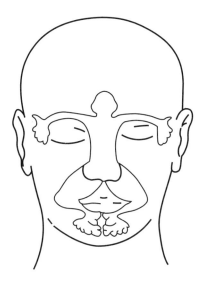

Illustration: *The original Vietnamese map: 'The Physical Body'*

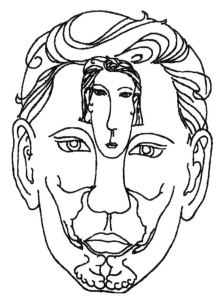

Illustration: *The original Vietnamese map of 'Hemispheres'*

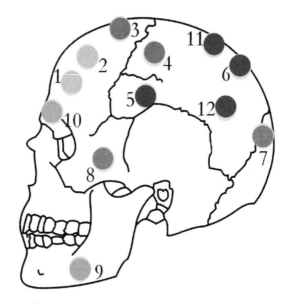

Illustration: *A map of the cranial points, based on cranial acupressure*

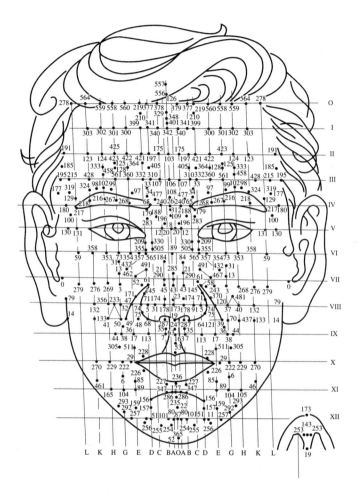

Illustration: *The Vietnamese map of the 564 neurological points*

In 1991, in a conference on 'Temprana Therapy', stimulation in Cordoba, Argentina, I studied the work of a French doctor, **Dr Jean Bossy**, which maps the interconnections between Oriental meridianology and the central nervous system. With the help of this knowledge, I completed my neurological map for feet and hands.

In the years that followed, I participated in and presented facial reflexology at various conferences in Latin America organized by the '**Dr Filipe Piñel Foundation**' in *Buenas Aires*. The foundation aims to investigate therapies to help and treat disabled children. In one of the conferences, I learnt about the methods of **Dr Castillo Morales**, an Argentinian specializing in facial and oral rehabilitation. After years of experience, **Dr Morales**, had created a manual muscle stimulation of the face with connections to the points and zones of the face. A part of the method is compatible with facial reflexology.

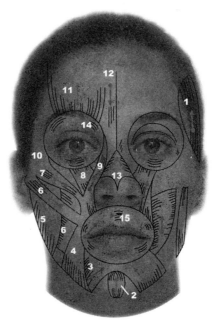

CHAPTER 3

Concept of Facial Reflexology

Skin is an organ of our body, which is subjected to more aggressions than any other organ, internally and externally. The ageing of the skin is chronological, irreversible and visual. The aggression of the internal and external influences can be controlled. Environmental factors such as – excessive consumption of carbohydrates and fats, exposure to sunlight, too little sleep, mental and physical stress, and ingestion of toxic substances such as coffee, alcohol and tobacco are some of the most common aggressions, which eventually reflect on the face. But before it reflects on face, the aggression has started a process which internally undermines the skin. As a secondary effect it appears as an external weakness and the skin breaks out, resulting in symptoms like flaky tissue, deep wrinkles, lack of collagen and elastin etc.

Facial Reflexology is a modern therapeutic method which is effective and uses manual stimulation. With the use of these methods, it is possible to alleviate the external influences and the biological deficiencies that appear on the face. Using the same therapy, it is also possible to stimulate points and reflex zones on the face to achieve a state of equilibrium in the body by affecting the organic physiology, the circulatory system, lymphatic system, etc. Facial reflexology also helps emotional symptoms such as – anguish, mental lethargy, memory loss, insomnia, etc. Facial Reflexology can be applied as a holistic and preventive treatment. Facial Reflexology also works as a post-surgical treatment, regulating the regenerative processes of wounds and also the organic influences produced by the surgery itself or by anesthetics. It is a natural technique, free of toxins and is very relaxing.

Facial Reflexology is an auxiliary therapy that actually has its origin in ancient Oriental medicine. It was later researched and modified by European and American doctors. Facial Reflexology has several stages. Seven basic zonal treatments allow the therapist to make a thorough assessment of the face for signs of diagnostic conditions, which will be different for each patient.

At the same time, a stimulation of the neuro-biological system and the central nervous system is performed by pressing specific points along meridians and on zones stimulating the blood flow. As a primary effect, deep relaxation is produced in the muscular system as well as in the nervous system.

It is important to understand the embroyonic relationship between the ectoderm and its derivative tissues, through which the central nervous system and the skin acquire an intrinsic and very close relationship, useful for Facial Reflexology.

So far we can say that there exists a cutaneous-nervous reflex initiated by the manual stimulation of points and specific zones or areas. Through the reticular formation, the impulse affects other segments of the peripheral and the vegetative nervous system, reaching skeletal muscles, articulations, bones, etc., and further reaches the organs and visceras. This means that a particular pressure on specific facial point or zone, will have an effect on the neuromotor and the neuro-vegetative system, in a unique way. Facial Reflexology is a method which can be used to maintain health and as an excellent preventive for diseases. This is evident by the fact that many sign can be detected on the zones of the face at an early stage giving the practitioner an idea about the health situation of a person. So, there is no need to have a verified specific pathology to enjoy a facial reflexology treatment. Everyday, more and more permutations and combinations of diseases of unknown etiology are discovered. The cause can be traced to stress, anxiety, anguish, frustration, etc. Therefore, this is a therapy that stimulates the whole nervous system resulting in a deep sedating effect, which is sustained for a long period of time and increases proportionally after a certain number of treatments. It is not necessary to be suffering a particular pathology to have a reflexology treatment.

Facial Reflexology responds to musculo-skeletal pains, such as bursitis, arthritis, fibrosis and reflex-muscular spasm caused by trauma. Great results have been achieved in cases of lithiasis of the kidneys and the gall bladder, and with the many types of headaches, depending on the etiology in each case.

There is also a biofeedback effect, so that patients can learn to control in a conscious manner pains, tensions, migraines, lumbar pain, etc. It has been proved that Reflexology acts on pain, which has a psychological origin.

Reflexology is a holistic treatment which acts on the whole body, balances the metabolism, the organic working, the muscular symmetry and activates the micro-circulation.

> **Facial Reflexology therapy can be defined as a reflex technique based on the neuro-biochemical action that is caused by stimulating an area or a point and which has both a general and/or partial effect on the entire organism.**

CHAPTER 4

Neurobiological Theory

By exploring the tissue in the zones of the face, it is possible to feel swellings, which are known as deposits. These deposits are found under the dermis. A deposit reflects an imbalance in an organ represented by that zone in the face.

Dr Jesús Manzanares, practising in Sagrada Familia Hospital in Barcelona carried out biopsies on skin tissues containing deposits. Studies revealed that the deposits are formed due to trauma in the connective tissue of the dermis, and he observed an accumulation of an abnormal percentage of water and fibre in the tissue.

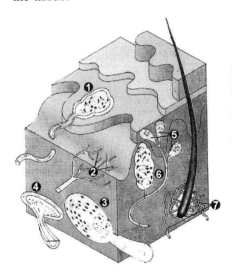

Stratification of the skin receptors:
1. Krause's bulbs
2. Free nerve ending
3. Pacini's bodies
4. Ruffini's bodies
5. Disk of Merkel
6. Meissner's bodies
7. Nerve ending of the hair follicles

Illustration: A cross section of the skin

In a square centimetre of skin there are twelve sebaceous glands, one hundred sweat glands, 2.5 metres of nerves, one metre of blood vessels and three million cells. The skin is the only external organ of the body. The skin acts as a defence system for the body from both inside and outside. The skin is also an important sensory organ relaying information about the external environment to the brain.

Grade (I) consistency of sand

Grade (II) consistency of small lumps

Grade (III) inflamation

Grade (IV) a moveable knot

Grade (V) an immovable knot

Illustration: Physical characteristics of the deposits

To be able to recognize deposit, the touch has to be very thorough in order to determine the levels affected. Study successively the following levels: cutaneous level, the muscular layer and the ligaments and bones.

By using two fingers, placing each of them in opposite direction and pulling them firmly away from each other, over the skin tissue, one is able to determine the grade of deposit in each area.

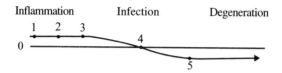

Illustration: A curve showing the development and formation of a deposit

Deposits in the area of the face indicate imbalance. The physical and the chemical agressions everyday on us are enough to cause the formation of deposits.

There are also other factors that influence the formation of deposits:

1. Usage of medicines
2. Serious illness affecting various organs
3. Emotional state—levels of stress and depression
4. The age of a patient

A powerful response achieved through Facial Reflexology, by stimulating the points and areas, can be explained as a change in the polarity of the cell. The cells which make up the tissue in the deposit have a negative electrical charge of 70 mV. In order to effect a change in the polarity of the cell through an impulse, manual stimulation is necessary.

Achieving an intense reflexological stimulus in the cell produces an increase in the electrical charge, up to +45mV. This is made possible by the entry of a larger quantity of ions: Na^+, K^+ Ca^+ into the cell.

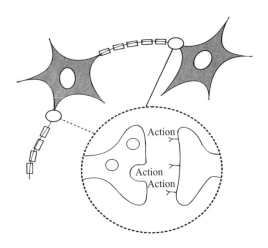

Illustration: A cellular electrical charge

Stimulating an area of the body, in principle, results in a rapid depolarization at a cellular level, followed by a phase of repolarization and lastly a phase of hyperpolarization. It is therefore, important and necessary to ensure that the stimulation is intensive (1 minute for each point), to be sufficient to achieve a powerful result.

Variations of the electrical charge

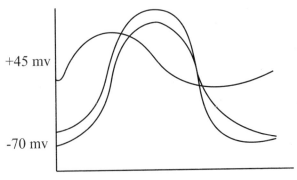

Illustration: The reaction of a cellular electricity charge during stimulation

The way of analyzing and identify deposits on a zone should be carried out in the direction recommended as shown below.

It is important to press firmly into the tissue but not to cause discomfort, especially around the area of the eyes.

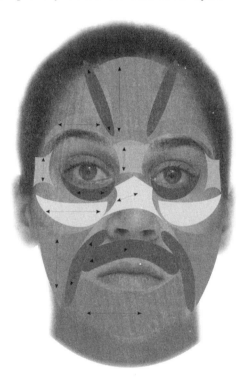

Illustration: *Reflexology zones on the face, used to stimulate and to analyze the state of health of a patient*

The intensity and number of sittings required for treatment varies from person to person depending on their physical, organic and emotional state of health including stress, anxiety, depression, etc. Other influencing factors include diet and medication.

CHAPTER 5

Technique in Practice

AFTER THE FIRST TREATMENT

After a treatment, it is natural for a patient to have certain reactions. These are signs that the body is responding to the treatment. The most common reactions are:

1. Tiredness
2. Tickling sensation
3. Temporary feelings of discomfort
4. Dizziness
5. Nausea
6. Frequent need to urinate
7. Strong smelling urine
8. Aches
9. Shivers
10. Perspiration

After the treatment, patients are advised to take a rest for 10-15 minutes and drink water to keep well hydrated. If a patient is taking medicine he/she must not stop taking it without consulting their doctor. The treatment should be carried out with the patient lying down comfortably upon a therapeutic couch/table. Facial Reflexology is suitable for everyone and at all ages. The duration of the treatment can vary depending on the patient's response. A typical session lasts between 45-60 minutes. It is a good practice to check the medical history of each patient.

> *The use of natural products (oils and creams) during treatment is recommended.*

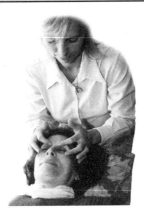

STEPS INVOLVED IN TECHNIQUE

Step 1– NP Points

The NP points on the face are stimulated using the hands. These points are directly related to the nerves of the central nervous system, the capillaries of microcirculation at a local level and to the meridians.

It is important that the stimulation is carried out using the tips of the second or middle finger and that the other fingers don't touch the face.

The treatment begins with the NP points on the chin and then moving up the face. Apart from those points that fall along the length of the central meridian, each point is mirrored on either side of the face and stimulated simultaneously. Eight to ten rotations with the fingertips should be given in clockwise direction. The points along the central meridian receive the same eight to ten rotations, but in both a clockwise and anticlockwise direction. This is because they are not repeated on both sides of the face.

These points are called neurovascular / NP points and when the electric flow of the nerve and of the meridian are not blocked, it is possible to feel a pulse. This is helpful when evaluating the effect of the treatment.

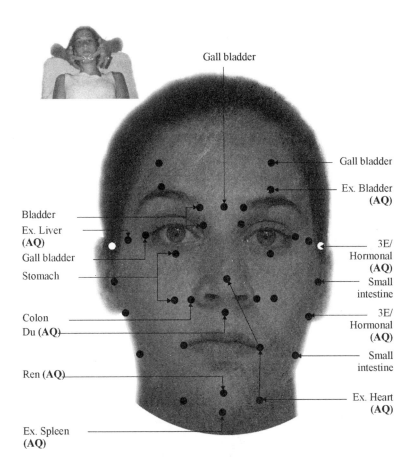

Gall bladder

Gall bladder

Ex. Bladder (AQ)

Bladder

Ex. Liver (AQ)

Gall bladder

Stomach

3E/ Hormonal (AQ)

Small intestine

Colon

Du (AQ)

3E/ Hormonal (AQ)

Small intestine

Ren (AQ)

Ex. Heart (AQ)

Ex. Spleen (AQ)

Illustration: *Ex. (AQ) points– points that are found in a meridian's ramification*

Step 2– The South American Indian Map

In step 2, the zones of the face are worked with deep movements pressing and stretching the tissue with long and smooth movements. These zones, which are used till date by South American Indian tribes, consist of nerve endings of the central nervous system. If there is a block in the nerve it will prevent the energy of the nerve impulse from flowing freely. In the nerve ending, underneath the dermis, a deposit of nerve fibers will be formed which will prevent the blood from circulating (the 5 stages of deposit). It is these deposits that can be felt while touching the face. Each zone has a network of nerves related and connected with the organs of the body. It is possible not only to determine the state of these vital organs that is, if they are functioning properly or not but also the state of health of the muscles, tendons, brain centre, glands secreting hormones, different chemical processes of the body, etc. since they are all connected with the zones of the vital organs via meridians.

While performing step 2 and working on all the zones, the biggest deposit must be found. This will define the meridian/zone to be treated in step 3.

These zones are to be stimulated equally on both sides of the face. It does not matter on which side the work begins.

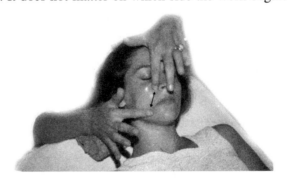

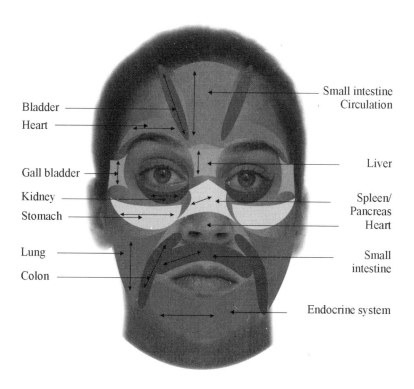

Small intestine
Circulation

Bladder

Heart

Liver

Gall bladder

Kidney

Spleen/
Pancreas
Heart

Stomach

Lung

Small
intestine

Colon

Endocrine system

Illustration: *Step 2– The South American Indian Map*

Step 3– The Vietnamese Map

Step 3 is the Vietnamese map of the face, showing the zones related to the meridians. This procedure is a deeper stimulation of the zone related to the biggest deposit in step 2 and the meridian pair associated with this biggest deposit. Small movements are used for 3 minutes.

All zones only have to be stimulated if the biggest deposit is in the hormonal area in Step 2.

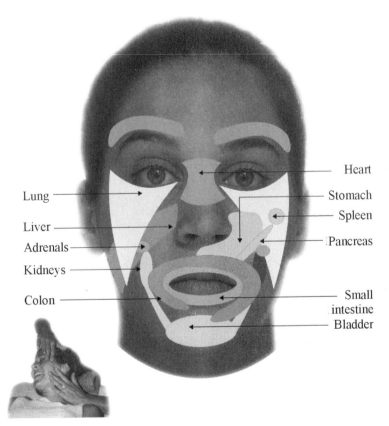

Illustration: *The hormonal and circulatory systems are activated by 11 zones*

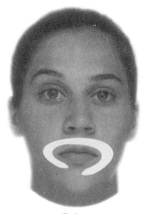

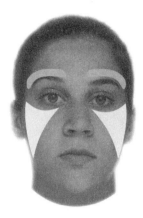

Colon   with   The Lungs

Lu: Lung
Co: Colon

St: Stomach
S/P :Spleen/Pancreas

H: Heart
SI: Small intestine

K: Kidney
B: Bladder

3E: Hormonal
C: Circulation

Li: Liver
Gb: Gall bladder

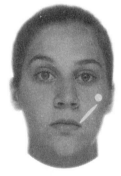

The Spleen and The Pancreas with

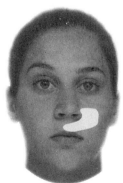

The Stomach

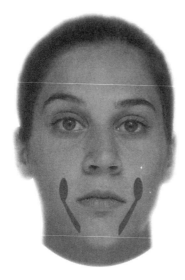

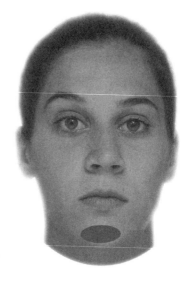

The Kidney   with   The Bladder

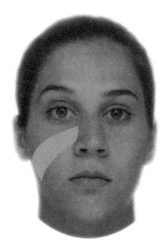
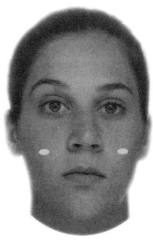

The Liver   with   The Adrenal glands

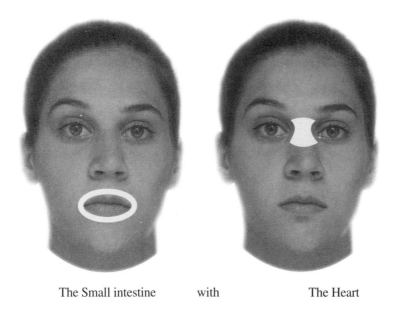

The Small intestine	with	The Heart

Illustration: *Zone related with meridian*

Step 4– Vietnamese Map

In step 4, the zones are related to the cortex of the brain and the cranial nerves. The Vietnamese map corresponds to the 12 cranial nerves of the sensory and motor cortex of the brain. As in step 3, these zones are treated with deep pressing and stretching of the tissue with short movements for 2-3 minutes. Begin on the area between the eyebrows - N° 6. Continue working up until the hairline - N° 1. Then to the right and down to the temple, down to the side of the face to under the ear - N° 14. Repeat the stimulation on the other side of the face in the same way.

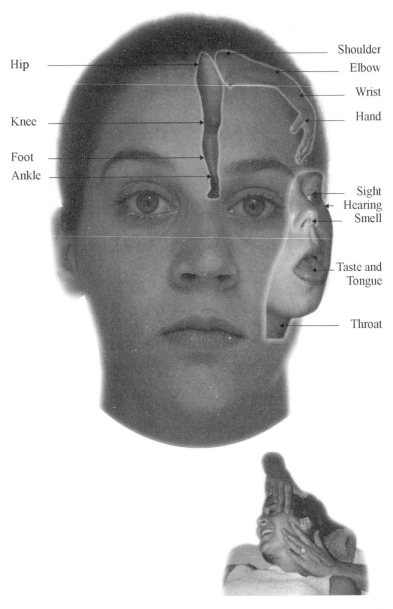

Hip

Shoulder
Elbow
Wrist
Hand

Knee

Foot
Ankle

Sight
Hearing
Smell

Taste and
Tongue

Throat

Illustration: *Vietnamese map corresponds to the 12 cranial nerves of the sensory and motor cortex of the brain*

Step 5– Vietnamese Map

In Step 5, the muscles, tendons, joints and spinal cord are stimulated by using the zonal map of the body. This is particularly beneficial to treat all kinds of problems of muscles and joints in the body. Like in step 3, these zones are treated using deep pressing and stretching of the tissue with short intensive movements.

Begin the treatment in the following manner:

1. The head

2. One of the arms

3. The other arm

4. The trunk

5. One of the legs and foot

6. The other leg and foot

Working intensively on the thin nasal wall achieves a direct stimulation upon the spinal cord.

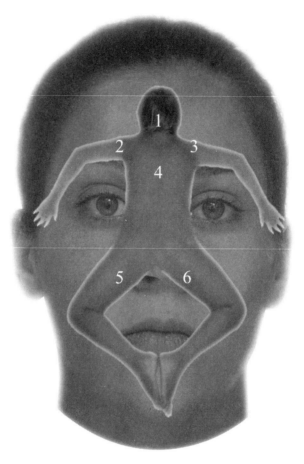

Illustration: *Step 5– Vietnamese map*

Illustration: *Working intensively on the thin nasal wall achieves a direct stimulation upon the spinal cord*

Step 6– NP Points

Step 6 is similar to step 1, which means the same NP points, are to be stimulated in the same order but this time with four rotations and four pumping pressure on each point. The aim is to achieve a lymphatic drainage effect.

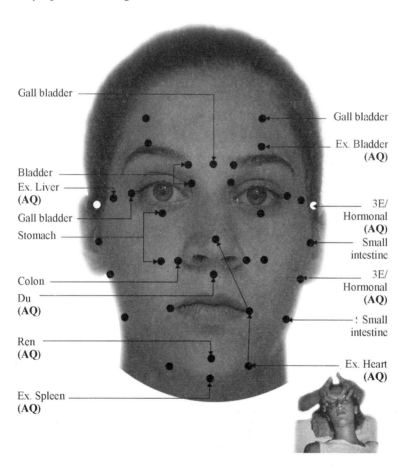

Illustration: *Step 6– NP points*

Step 7– Vietnamese Map

Make circular movements using the thumbs, beginning with the area of the brain on the forehead, then descend down the wall of the noseflare out to the cheeks until the area between the nose and mouth is reached. One by rubbing the lower part **(AQ)** of the chin. This cycle should be repeated three times.

The aim of step 7 is to balance the brain hemispheres and the areas of the brain that deal with the coordination, making it possible to regain a better balance and function of coordination between the hemispheres.

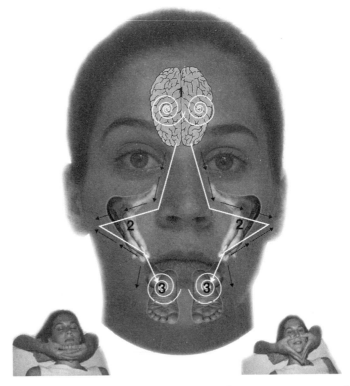

Illustration: *Step 7– Vietnamese map. Circular movements are made moving down from forehead to chin*

The 7 steps that make up the basic treatment

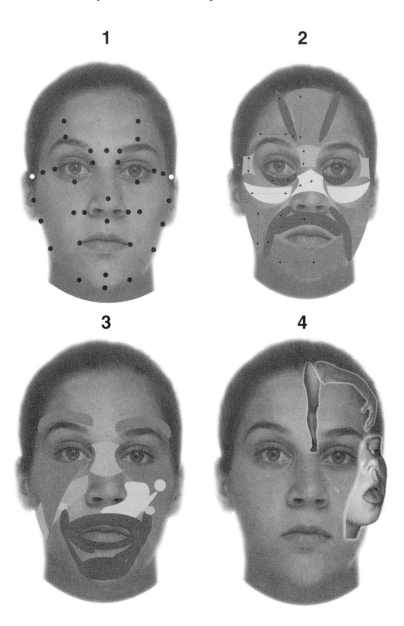

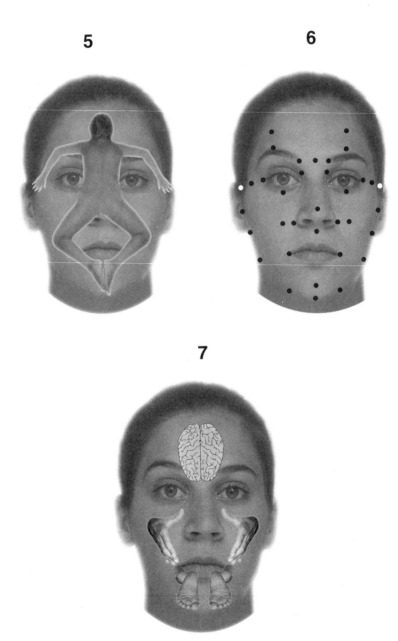

Illustration: *The seven steps which make up the basic treatment*

The 7 steps that make up the basic treatment

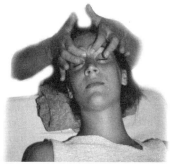

1. The NP points

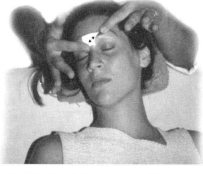

2. The South American Indian zones

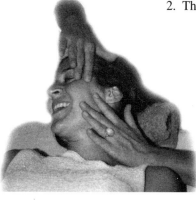

3. Vietnamese zones

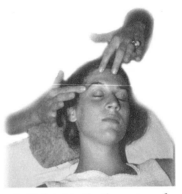

4. Related to the the cortex of
the brain

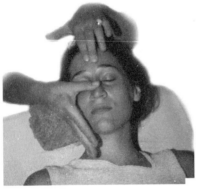

5. Zones for Vietnamese
'physical body'

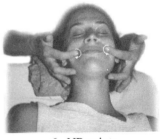

6. NP points

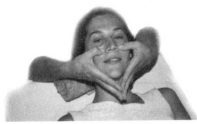

7. Vietnamese The 'psychological body'

Products Used for Therapy

It is important that the products used should be free from colorants, preservatives and other chemical components since these are absorbed by the skin and can produce unpleasant biochemical reactions.

It is recommended that natural creams or oils should be used. However, they can have side effects too.

It is recommended to use following aromatherapy oils for patients with large deposits in the following zones:

Large intestine, Heart, Blood, circulation and Hormonal - Dry skin:
Rosemary, Ylang-Ylang, Pachouli and Orange.

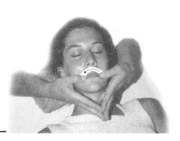

Stomach, Pancreas, Spleen - Oily skin:

Lemon

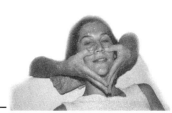

Lung, Colon - Fragile skin:
Pine and Cypress.

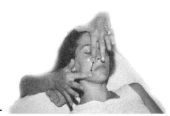

Liver, gall bladder - Acne
Lavender, Grapefruit and Thyme.

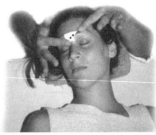

Kidneys, bladder - Sensitive skin:
Jasmine and Sandalwood.

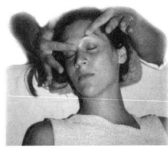

For all skin types it is possible to use Rose Hip Oil as base oil, adding essential oils.

CHAPTER 6

Conduction of the Impulse Through the Nervous System

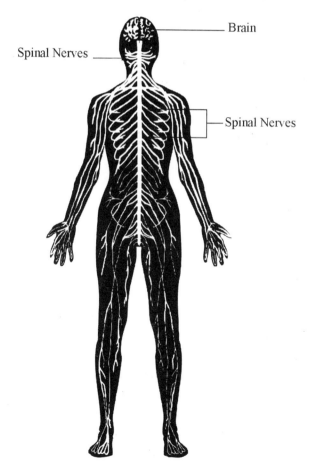

Illustration: *The nervous system*

The nervous system is composed of:

1.   Central nervous system (CNS)
2.   Peripheral nervous system (PNS)
3.   Autonomic nervous system (ANS)

CENTRAL NERVOUS SYSTEM (CNS)

CNS is composed of the brain and spinal cord.

Functions

CNS is the mediator between the outside world and our inner world. It makes every function in our system possible. It controls body functions and structures by keeping the body in balance (homeostasis).

PERIPHERAL NERVOUS SYSTEM (PNS)

PNS is composed of:

1.   12 pairs of cranial nerves
2.   31 pairs of spinal nerves

These are the motor, sensory fibers as well as the mixed fibres (nerves). The spinal cord is a direct downward continuation of the brain stem that starts at the upper border of the first vertebra (called the atlas) and ends at the lower border of the first lumbar vertebra.

The peripheral nervous system (PNS) is basically an extension of the central nervous system. The peripheral nervous system connects the central nervous system with all the tissues of body. The 31 pairs of spinal nerves is a very complex network of nerves reaching out to every part of the body. Messages or signals to/from these nerves form a relay from the tissues of the body back to the brain and vice versa.

AUTONOMIC NERVOUS SYSTEM (ANS)

The autonomic nervous system (ANS), also known as the 'involuntary' nervous system controls activities of the body unconsciously. The autonomic nervous system includes all the nerve cells or neurons, located outside the spinal cord and the brain stem.

The ANS itself is divided into two separate entities: the Sympathetic and the Parasympathetic divisions. The sympathetic division sends impulses that speed up or enhance life processes and vital function whereas the parasympathetic slows down the same. These two systems together regulate the majority of the body's involuntary functions. Examples of involuntary control are the heart beat, respiration, blood circulation and digestion.

Spinal Cord

The spinal cord is a cylinder of nerve tissue that runs down the central canal in the spine. The nerve fibers in the spinal cord transmit sensory information towards the brain and motor signals to the appropriate part of the body. The spinal cord itself also handles some automatic motor responses to sensory information.

The Central nervous system, composed of the brain and spinal cord is a system that regulates body functions like thinking, behaviour, motor and sensory activity, and through which facial reflexology works.

In the CNS, there are important areas like Neo cortex, the limbic system and diverse systems that interact with one another making vital functions in the body like blood circulation, hormone releasing and thinking possible.

The PNS, is composed of 12 pairs of cranial nerves and 31 pairs of spinal nerves. The 12 pairs of cranial nerves originate from the brain and innervate muscles which control the movement of the eyes or the swallowing function, and facial movements. Some of them have sensory functions such as the olfactory or the optic nerves which help in smelling and vision.

There are also mixed nerves, which have both motor and sensory fibers, like the trigeminal nerve that gives sensitivity to the face but also helps movement of the lower jaw.

The 31 pairs of spinal nerves come out of the gaps between the vertebrae and innervate different organs like the stomach, heart, lungs, liver etc. helping them to function.

The nervous system is formed by highly specialized cells called neurons, which are responsible for transmitting impulses by means of chemicals called neurotransmitters, like serotonin and dopamine, among others.

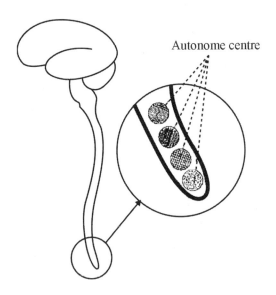

Autonome centre

Illustration: The spinal cord is a nervous structure which is found inside the back bone

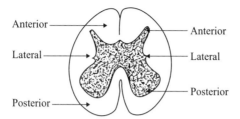

Illustration: A cross section of the spinal cord. The grey substance is shaped like wings, neurons are found in this grey matter

The Nerve System

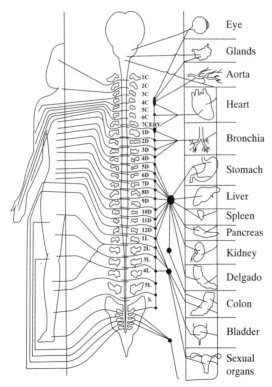

Illustration: The structures which drive the reflex impulse to the spinal cord are called sensory nerves. They control sensation and are ending within the face area

In the picture we can see the sensory territory of each nerve in the body.

The Twelve Pairs of Cranial Nerves

The 12 pairs of cranial nerves with functions are:

I.   Olfactory – Smell

II. Optic – Vision

III. Oculomotor – Eyelid and eyeball movements

IV. Trochlear – Innervates superior and oblique muscles of eyes, turns eye downward and laterally

V.   Trigeminal – Chewing, sensory fibres of face and mouth helping in touch and pain

VI. Abducens – Turns eye laterally

VII. Facial – Controls most facial expressions, secretion of tears and saliva, taste sensation

VIII. Vestibulocochlear / auditory – Hearing, and maintaining equilibrium and balance

IX. Glossopharyngeal – Taste sensation of tongue, controls blood pressure

X.   Vagus – Taste, slows heart rate and stimulates digestive organs

XI. Spinal Accessory – Controls trapezius and sternocleido-mastoid muscles and controls swallowing movements

XII. Hypoglossal – Controls movements of tongue

Relationship Between the Cranial Nerves and the NP Points

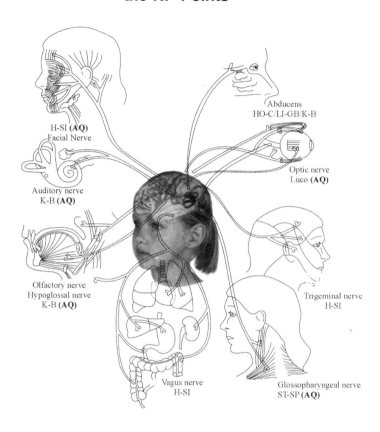

Illustration: Relationship between the cranial nerves and the NP points

APPENDIX: NEUROVASCULAR POINTS

The following pages list symptoms arising from cranial nerve dysfunction and the NP point to use.

Press on the two NP points that belong to the nerve you want to treat, 1 minute at the same time.

Anatomical Connection: Co 20
The facial veins and arteries and the parafacial orbital nerve.

Indications:
Facial paralysis
Sinusitus
Dental (crooked teeth)
Facial edema
Nasal polyps
Nasal hemorrhage

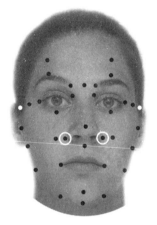

Illustration: Anatomical connection: Co 20 (AQ)

Anatomical Connection: GB 14
The branches of the frontal veins and arteries and the branches of the frontal nerves.

Indications:
Frontal headaches
Contracture of the neck
Headache
Spasms of the eye muscle
Migraines
Eyelid tics
Vertigo

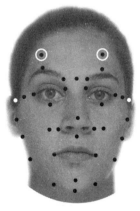

Illustration: Anatomical Connection: GB 14

Anatomical Connection: 3E/Ho 22
Temporal vein and artery
Branches of the auriculotemporal,
temporal and facial nerve.

Indications:
Headache
Tension of the masseter muscle
Heaviness in the head
Facial paralysis
Tinnitus

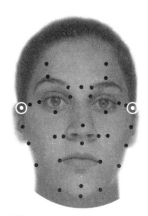

Illustration: Anatomical
connection: 3E/Ho 22

Anatomical Connection: GB-1
Zygomatic facial veins and arteries.
The branches of the temporal facial
nerves.

Indications:
Conjunctivitis
Eye strain
Headaches
Glaucoma
Red eyes and epiphora (tearing)
Sore throat

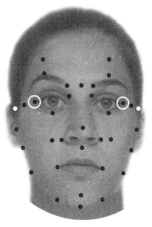

Illustration: Anatomical
connection: GB-1
Zygomatic facial veins
and arteries

**Anatomical – Neurological
Connection:** St1-2-3x. St.
Ramifications of the arteries,
infraorbital vein and ocular vein.
Front ramifications of the
oculomotor facial nerve.

Indications:
Strabismus
Atrophy of the optic nerve
Conjunctivitis
Eyelash spasms
Constant flow from the tear ducts
Pressure in the eyes
Myopia
Cataract
Facial paralysis
Deviation of the corner of the mouth
Facial spasms
Allergies
Headache
Pain in the face

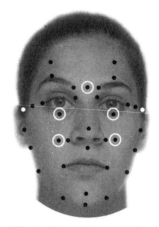

Illustration: Anatomical –
Neurological Connection:
St1-2-3x. St.

**Anatomical – Neurological
Connections:** B 1-2
The internal artery of the eye and
ophthalmia. Frontal vein,
infraorbital, supratrochlear, motor,
ocular and frontal nerves.

Indications:
Conjunctivitis
Cataract
Ocular pressure
Ocular hemorrhage
Decrease in sharpness of vision
Facial paralysis
Vertigo
Headache
Infant fits
Spasms of the eyelashes

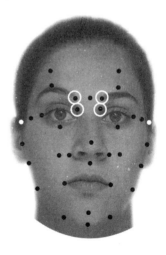

Illustration: Anatomical –
Neurological Connection:
B 1-2

Anatomical – Neurological Connection: Si 19

Superficial artery and veins. Facial and auriculotemporal nerves.

Indications:

Colic
Earache
Deviation of the teeth
Infections of the middle ear
Deafness
Muteness
Titinnus

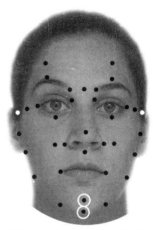

Illustration: Anatomical – Neurological Connection: Si 19

Anatomical – Neurological Connection: Cen. 24-25

Indications:

Labial artery and vein
Facial nerve
Mental confusion
Deviation of the mouth
Dental pain
Hemiplegia
Facial paralysis
Snoring
Excessive salivation

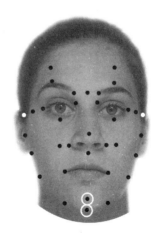

Illustration: Anatomical – Neurological Connection: Cen. 24-25

Anatomical – Neurological Connection:

Arterial and facial vein.
Facial nerve, infraorbitals and ramifications of the bucal nerve.

Indications:

Facial deviation
Deviation of the mouth
Eyelid spasms
Excessive salivation
Facial paralysis
Trigeminal neuralgia
Loss of voice

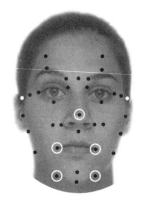

Illustration: Anatomical – Neurological Connection: Facial artery and vein

Anatomical – Neurological Connection:

Labial artery and vein. Bucal facial nerve and infraorbital nerve.

Indications:

Nasal congestion
Aphonia
Coma
Mental problems
Lumbar pain
Epilepsy
Infant fits
Spasms of the facial muscles
Facial paralysis
Thirst
Schizophrenia

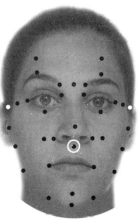

Illustration: Anatomical – Neurological Connection: Labial artery and vein

The nervous system is activated by possible informations and impulses from outside the body. The external impulses cause a reaction within the central nervous system. So it is logical to assume that a powerful internal reaction can be achieved possibly by external stimulation. These stimulations and impulses can be: pressure, light, sound, color, smell, heat and cold, etc.

Actions in Nervous System

External Impulses:

Vision	Movement
Hearing	Hormonal system
Touch	Respiration
Taste	Digestion

Internal Impulses:

Temperature	Circulatory
Arterial pressure	Eliminatory
Ph	Memory
Thought process	Development of constructive thinking

These actions are due to three different system:

1. The hormonal system
2. The peripheral nervous system
3. The central nervous system

Interpretation of The Pulses on The Points

After the basic stimulation has been carried out, it is possible to detect a pulse on the points. Pulse indicates that the electric impulse is flowing freely. There are situations when the pulses are only registered on one side of the face. This signifies that there is an imbalance in the electric current of the organism. It is important to use the radial pulse when interpreting what is going in the body because it can express emotional blockages.

The radial pulse is where you can perceive whether or not the body is in harmony. Pulse changes and varies constantly. However, its general characteristics don't change. There are three types of pulse:

1.   Nervous pulse
2.   Visceral-hormonal pulse
3.   Lymphatic pulse

Visceral-hormonal pulse – NP points

Visceral-hormonal pulse is characterized by its bluntness and the power of the pulse beats. They are very clear and sharp. Any mental tension or stress suffered by an individual tends to manifest itself on the digestive, hepatobiliary and hormonal area.

Nervous pulse – N points

Nervous pulse is the quickest and weakest pulse. The nervous pulse can be psychogenetic or transitory. It is seen in people who react very quickly to stressful situations. These are emotional type of people, who move rapidly from one state to another without a clear motive. They are very receptive to reflexology.

Any psychological problems suffered by these individuals tends to manifest itself on the nervous and respiratory system.

Lymphatic pulse, cranial points

Lymphatic pulse is a very slow pulse, weak and resistant, without a strong beat. The lymphatic pulse is seen in people who have difficulty in getting rid of psychological tension, which then has an impact on their organs of elimination and thus, the lymphatic system. The emotional 'knots' produce retention in the body in the form of:

1.   Water retention
2.   Organic swellings
3.   Retention of fatty materials

Depending on the grade and intensity of the affliction, there are several signs, which can be seen by simply observing the face. These are: the intensity of the color and complexion, congestion or discoloration with an increase in vascularization, moles, vitiligo, small nodules, open pores and small scars.

INDEX

Lu: Lung
Co: Colon
St: Stomach
S/P: Spleen/Pancreas
H: Heart
SI: Small intestine
K: Kidney
B: Bladder
3E: Hormonal
C: Circulation
L: Liver
Gb: Gall bladder
Cen: Central (Ren)
Gov: Governor (Du)

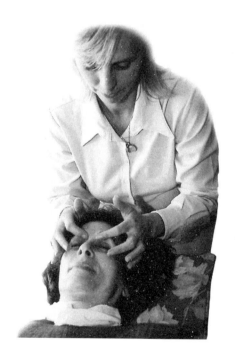

CHAPTER 7

Traditional Oriental Theory

Chinese medicine recognizes three circulatory networks in the human body: the nerves, the blood vessels and the energy meridians. Western medicine recognizes only the first two.

Traditional Chinese medicine asserts that the energy is sent to the blood. This means the blood circulates only through tissues where the energy flows freely. When the energy meridians are blocked, not enough blood circulates. The same principle applies to the nervous system. Chinese medicine recognizes that nervous as well as circulatory disorders, can be corrected with therapies such as acupuncture, which stimulates and balances the flow of energy around all the networks of meridians. Meridians form an invisible network which flows through the circulatory and nervous system in the body.

The three circulatory systems must be balanced and synchronized in order to maintain health. However, it is the network of the meridians and their subtle energy that has to be manipulated and restored in order to correct any problems within the three systems. In this way we can see that energy in Chinese medicine as the focal point of human health.

For at least five thousand years, the Chinese have known about the existence of a network of invisible human energy. They discovered that human energy flows through the body by means of a complex network of large canals, organs, meridians and small capillaries, throughout which a series of sensitive energy points are also found. These points act as transmission stations and transformers for the energy.

These points (each one of which produces specific effects upon the organs, certain tissues and upon the related energy) constitute the basis of acupuncture, moxibution and digit acupuncture therapies. The most powerful canals of the human energy network are the 8 extraordinary meridians which function like stores of energy for all the organisms and can be activated and replenished by the aforementioned therapies. (The 8 extraordinary meridians are not mentioned in this book.)

The principle meridians are the Governor and the meridian of Conception, which make up what is known as the **microcosmic**, and which give energy to the entire organism. Next, there are the twelve meridians which are associated with the twelve vital energy systems of the organs. These meridians pass like conductors through the entire organism, irrigating the organs, glands and tissues, giving them nutritive energy and managing their vital functions. They send energy to the main organ systems following a specific order. From the eight principal canals and the twelve meridians of the organs, an infinite number of small capillaries branch out and form a fine network, which provides energy to each cell in the body.

The network of human energy performs numerous functions. It regulates the circulation and blood pressure, maintains the external cortex of the protective energy of the body, intervenes in the nervous system, distributes nutritive energy to all the organism, controls body temperature, feeds the metabolism and establishes all the functional links between the body and the mind.

In Chinese medicine all pathology, physiology as well as mental and emotional problems are considered symptoms reflecting a serious imbalance and malfunctioning within the human energy network.

By using logic and thinking carefully it is possible to understand the Chinese system of energy distribution and to establish by whatever means possible, its relationship with the general theory of Chinese medicine. Chinese medicine implicates the idea of charging, supporting and transporting of the energetic current of the meridians.

In our times, the first extensive medicine compendium, the Huangdi Neijing dedicated an extensive part to physiology and the pathology of these 'canals', called meridians through which vital energy circulates.

The meridians have a habitual internal route passing through the organs and viscera, as well as a superficial external route which is what acupuncture is concerned with.

These meridians intervene in the control of the organic functions and can be classified in two groups: *ordinary* and *extraordinary*. The ordinary, twelve in number, are more well known than the extraordinary meridians which are eight.

A direct relationship exists between the meridians and the diseases of certain organs. Each ordinary meridian carries the name of an organ, with the exception of the hormonal (triple heater) and circulation-sexual (pericardium) meridians and they subdivide into zang organs: solid and visceral, and fú hollow organs.

The zang organs are related with the 'yin' and the fú with the 'yang', and lastly they subdivide into:

The three yang meridians of the hand
The three yang meridians of the feet
The three yin meridians of the hand
The three yin meridians of the feet

Meridian	Yin-Yang	Limb	Hour of maximum activity
1. Lung	Yin	Ends in the body	3-5 a.m.
2. Large intestine	Yang	Begins in the hand	5-7 a.m.
3. Stomach	Yang	Ends in the foot	7-9 a.m.
4. Spleen/Pancreas	Yin	Ends in the hand	11-1 p.m.
5. Heart	Yin	Begins in the foot	9-11 a.m.
6. Small intestine	Yang	Begins in the hand	1-3 p.m.
7. Bladder	Yang	Ends in the foot	3-5 p.m.
8. Kidney	Yin	Begins in the foot	5-7 p.m.
9. Circulatory	Yin	Ends in the hand	7-9 p.m.
10. Hormonal	Yang	Begins in the hand	9-11 p.m.
11. Gall bladder	Yang	Ends in the foot	11-1 a.m.
12. Liver	Yin	Begins in the foot	1-3 a.m.

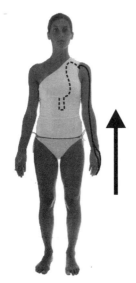

Lungs

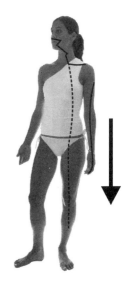

Colon

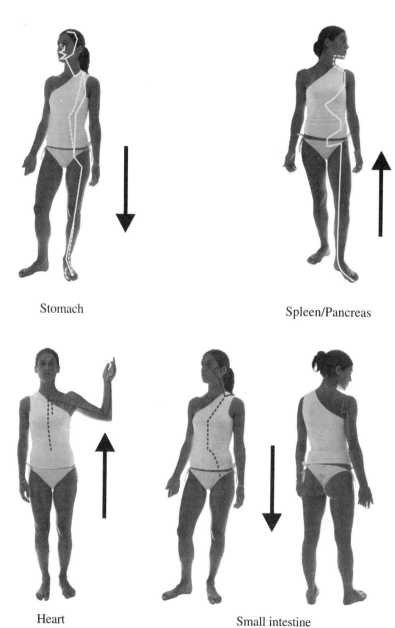

Stomach

Spleen/Pancreas

Heart

Small intestine

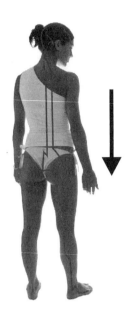

Bladder

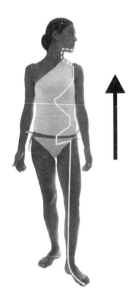

Kidney

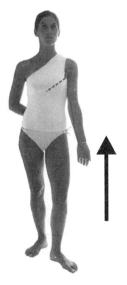

Circulatory

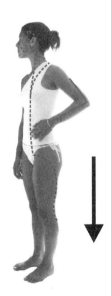

Hormonal

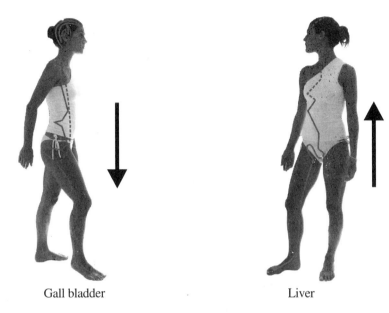

Gall bladder   Liver

Illustration*: Course of Yang meridians*

According to the classical / traditional theory, the energy circulates through the meridians in the order in which they are related: always beginning with the lung meridian which has its origin in the thorax and flows towards the hand. Here it connects with the meridian of the large intestine and returns to the upper limb, neck and face; from here it connects with the stomach via face and then descends towards the foot where it connects with the spleen meridian. Then it ascends towards the thorax and in the same way repeats the flow with the remaining meridians:

1. All the meridians that start in the hand are yang and those that end in the hand are yin.
2. All the meridians that start in the foot are yin and those that end in the foot are yang.
3. The three yin hand meridians start in the thorax and end in the hand.

4. The three yang meridians in the hand begin in the hand and end in the face.

5. The three yang meridians in the foot begin in the face and end in the foot.

6. The three yin meridians begin in the foot and end in the thorax.

The current flows from the chest towards the hands passing through the three yin meridians in the arm: the lung, circulation and heart meridians. Here the aforementioned meridians connect with the three yang meridians which go to make up their pair, the lung, the endocrine which partners the circulation meridian and lastly the small intestine respectively and go down right to the feet where they connect to the corresponding yin: spleen, liver and kidneys, and then return towards the chest to complete the cycle.

Despite the fact that the current circulates continually through the twelve regular meridians there are moments when the flux of energy and blood reach a culminating point in a meridian. The maximum daily quota of the flow of energy in each meridian is shown next (the hours of maximum activity are shown on the previous page).

FUNCTIONS OF THE MERIDIANS

Meridians are the structures that join the flow of energy throughout the body. They connect interior to the exterior and are passages of concentrations of energy and blood, which run through the body. Their function is to transport the energy around the body. Though it may sound contradictory at times, they are the access routes for the pathogenic factors that invade the body first externally then internally. The meridians supply the points of entrance for the energy flow.

THE COMMUNICATION BETWEEN THE MERIDIANS

The meridians in the arms and legs are connected to each other. The problem that appears in certain meridians or organs can be treated using the points of the connected meridian.

For example, a lung disorder can be treated through certain acupuncture points corresponding to the spleen meridian because both are yin meridians.

Each meridian is connected to its corresponding organ. This is a clear example of internal/external communication. In the same way, each yin meridian is connected to its corresponding yang meridian and vice versa.

For example:

1.   A problem in the colon meridian can be treated by working on the acupuncture points of the lung meridian as well as the colon meridian, lung is the partner.

2.   A problem with the kidneys can be treated by working on the acupuncture points of not only the kidney but the bladder as well because the bladder is the yang partner of the kidneys.

It is important to realise that the disease of an organ can affect the corresponding organs by means of the meridian system.

THE NETWORK OF MERIDIANS

The main distributory vessels of blood are the arteries and the veins, but a large number of connecting capillaries which ensure the circulation of blood throughout the body are also important. In the same way, the meridian system is made up of a network consisting of small connecting branches.

The Fifteen Connectory Meridians

These meridians connect the yin and yang canals. For example, the heart meridian with the colon meridian.

Each of the twelve major channels connect a meridian, the spleen meridian has two and the governor and the central meridians have one each, which in total makes fifteen meridians.

YIN AND YANG

According to the ancient theory, yin and yang are two opposed forces, present throughout nature. One cannot exist without the other and nothing is totally yin or totally yang. When an imbalance occurs between the two, one of the two will predominate resulting in illness of whatever proportion whether it be a mild symptom or something more severe.

Functions of the Yang Meridian

Colon meridian

The colon absorbs the pure and excretes the impure. It receives the impurities from the small intestine, refines them to extract any remaining liquid or pure essence available and excretes the impurities in the form of feces. The colon is paired with the lungs.

Stomach meridian

The stomach receives and stores food. Thereafter it separates the important part and passes it to the spleen where it is refined and converted into energy, the rest is sent to the small intestine, if the stomach does not complete its function of sending energy in the downward direction for processing, it rises upwards and provokes hiccups, nausea and vomiting. The stomach is paired with the spleen.

Small intestine meridian

The small intestine's function is to separate the pure from the impure. The small intestine receives partially digested food from the stomach. The pure part is extracted by the spleen and the impure passes to the large intestine or bladder to be excreted. The small intestine performs similar function with fluids. The small intestine is paired with the heart.

Bladder meridian

The bladder stores urine and controls its excretion. The bladder receives any spare body fluids coming from the lungs, small intestine and large intestine under the influence and control of the kidneys. It stores them and excretes them in the form of urine. The bladder is paired with the kidneys.

Triple heater/Hormonal

The triple heater meridian coordinates the transformation and transportation of fluids. It coordinates the flow of water to the upper, middle and lower body. It can be compared to a director supervising his team. It regulates the working of body and controls the coordination of energy from the kidneys, moving it around and maintaining the temperature of the body. The triple heater is also known as the hormonal meridian. The triple heater meridian is paired with the pericardium.

Gall bladder meridian

The gall bladder stores bile. The bile is stored and excreted in the digestive tract to help facilitate digestion. The gall bladder dominates our capacity to take decisions. The gall bladder controls our ability to judge and be reasonable. Its malfunction can stop us from taking correct decisions. The gall bladder is paired with the liver.

Functions of the Yin Meridians

Lung meridian

The lung meridian governs the lungs and breathing. During inhalation, the lungs take in oxygen from the universe and turn it into energy in the body and during exhalation they expel carbon dioxide from the body. The lungs are very sensitive to emotional feelings and turmoil. Excessive sadness and grief can lead to imbalances and illness in the lungs. The lungs are also sensitive to changes in the environment such as wind, dampness and coldness. There is very little protection in the air we breathe which leaves our lungs susceptible to imbalances.

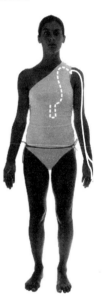

Illustration: *Course of lung meridian*

Spleen meridian

Spleen regulates transport and conversion

The spleen extracts nutrients from food in the stomach and transports them to the lungs and heart for conversion into energy and blood. A healthy spleen is reflected in a healthy appetite and a strong digestion, energy and a healthy muscle tone. Dysfunction of the spleen manifests itself in symptoms of tiredness, abdominal distension, bad digestion and diarrhea.

Spleen holds the blood

The function of the spleen is to control the flow of blood inside the blood vessels. A dysfunctioning spleen can cause loss of blood, which reflects in the form of blood in stool and urine or as a tendency to bruise easily.

Spleen dominates the muscles and the extremities

The spleen transports energy across the body and assures the shape and correct tone of the muscles. Any type of energy deficiency in the spleen causes bad muscle tone which translates into fatigue, weight loss and a weak and lax musculature.

Spleen controls energy

Most important function of the spleen is to exert an elevatory effect upon the internal organs. An imbalance in the working of the spleen can cause problems such as internal prolapse and diarrhea.

Spleen controls thought

Spleen sends clean energy to the head and brain. The ability to think clearly and to concentrate depends upon the proper working of the spleen. An upset in the spleen provokes a deficiency in clean energy to the head, which in its turn means confusion and in some cases mental disorders.

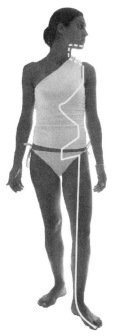

Illustration: *Course of spleen meridian*

Yin Meridians

Heart meridian

Heart regulates blood

Heart controls and regulates the flow of blood in blood vessels. It maintains a moderate temperature in the extremities and a constant and uniform pulse. Heart is also responsible for transforming energy from food into blood. It also intervenes in the ventilation of the lungs, strengthens the heart beat and gets the blood moving.

Heart controls the blood vessels

Proper working of blood vessels results in good circulation of blood, where as, dysfunction can lead to illness.

Heart maintains a healthy mental status

When the heart is under control, we can use the attributes of our personality in a constructive and healthy way, but if it is below par, a series of mental disorders and psychological disorders can appear. The state of the heart is reflected in the eyes.

Heart is manifested in the complexion

Rosy and radiant complexion indicates the heart is working properly or else the complexion appears dull and lifeless. If the malfunction is very serious, it can paralyze blood and skin can take on a blue tone.

The state of heart is reflected in the tongue

If the blood to the heart is insufficient the tongue will be pale and when the blood in the heart stagnates, the tongue appears purple in color.

Heart controls perspiration

The blood and body fluids share the same origin and there is a continuous exchange going on between them.

The heart keeps us happy

The way in which a person manifests his happiness in an appropriate way will reflect the state of health of the heart.

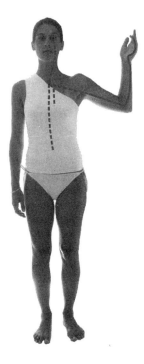

Illustration: Course of heart meridian

Kidney meridian

Kidneys store vital energy and control reproduction, development and growth

The vital energy is stored in the kidneys, which are responsible for growth and development during infancy. They are also a fundamental factor in ensuring that sexual and reproductive functions are normal. Any problem with the energy in kidneys can lead to delayed growth, learning difficulties, sterility, sexual problems and premature senility.

Kidneys make marrow, shape the brain, control bones and make blood

The energy emanating from kidneys is responsible for the production of marrow (an essential element of the bones), bone marrow, spinal cord and the structure of the brain. So, for the bones and teeth to be strong and healthy, and brain to function properly, kidneys need to be kept healthy. A problem in the production of marrow can cause ringing in the ears, blurred vision, mental problems and pain in the lumbar region. Moreover, marrow is involved in the production of blood.

A decline in the smooth functioning of kidney can be associated with insufficient production of blood.

Kidneys regulate water

Kidneys control the lower energy. Its other functions are the elimination of residual water from the body. When kidneys function well, the clean fluids are sent to the lungs and the dirty fluids are excreted through the bladder or else urinary problems may occur.

Kidneys emerge in our sense of hearing

Any kind of infection and malfunctioning of kidneys results in hearing problem.

Kidneys reveal themselves in the state of the hair

When they function well, the hair will be healthy and shiny and when they don't, the hair becomes fragile, lifeless and dull. It can also turn prematurely grey.

Kidneys control will power and fear

Kidneys are the basis of life and as a consequence, the perception of personal power and the will to succeed depends largely on the proper functioning of the kidneys. When they fail to function properly, a person may feel weak and shy resulting in the individual feeling incapable of facing a difficult life situations.

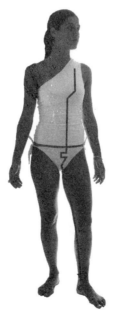

Illustration: *Course of Kidney meridian*

Pericardium/Circulatory meridian

The pericardium/circulatory are closely associated with the heart.

The pericardium/circulatory protects the heart

It is understood that the circulation as a whole, joins all external and visceral membranes, which surrounds and protects the heart. The pericardium protects the heart from pathogenic, external, invading agents and problems such as high fever. The pericardium retains the heat and in doing so protects the principle yin organ of the body, the heart.

The circulatory guides happiness and pleasure

Quietens the heart and produces feelings of happiness. As a protector of the heart, the pericardium acts as a guide throughout our lives helping us to experiment with happiness and pleasure in a balanced way.

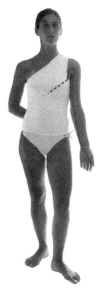

Illustration: Course of Circulatory meridian

Liver meridian

Liver stores the blood

The liver increases the flow of blood. When the body needs less blood flow, the liver is responsible for storing the excess until it is needed again. When the liver is healthy, the body receives a good supply of blood and is healthy, strong and flexible, whereas when there is disease, debility and rigidity occur.

Liver controls the uniform flow of energy

It is considered that the said functioning of the liver, of uniforming and giving fluidity is related to the harmonization of the emotions. Emotional blockages cause problems such as anger and frustration.

Liver controls the tendons

Tendons and ligaments are controled by liver. As such, the liver is considered very important when it comes to movement and flexibility. The capacity of the tendons to expand and contract in an effective way depends on the body receiving the correct nutrition needed to support the liver.

Liver manifests itself in the nails

If the liver's blood is healthy, then the nails will be strong and hydrated as compared to when there is insufficient blood to the liver which tends to make the nails thin, brittle and pale in color.

Healthy liver is a key to healthy eyes

It is thought that the state of health of the eyes depends on the proper functioning of the liver. When blood to the liver is insufficient, ocular problems occur.

The liver exerts control

When the liver is balanced and functions well, we can control the events happening in our lives and respond to unwanted changes in a reasonable and flexible manner. However, when the liver is in a state of dysfunction we become uncontrolable, rigid and inflexible or show a lack of control which is revealed in the form of excessive anger and irrational behavior.

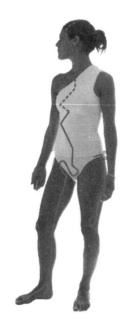

Illustration: Course of Liver meridian

Workings of the Extraordinary Du and Ren Meridians

They are similar to the Fu meridian as they are considered to be empty, although they perform storage functions, something which is more closely related to zang organs. They usually store the yin essentials of the body, the medulla and blood.

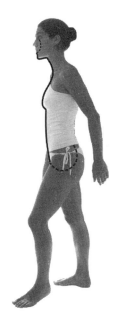 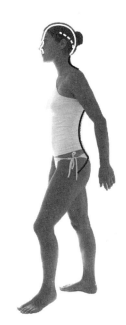

Illustration: The working of Cen and Gov meridians

CAUSES OF IMBALANCE

Once the elaborated system used by Chinese medicine to understand the body and its processes has been described, the importance of the idea of a dynamic balance within the system is obvious. On the other hand, Chinese medicine considers that illness is a result of influences that disturb harmony and balance, in all the energy system and although this influence may appear as specific symptoms, it is important not to loose sight of the balance of the whole.

We can divide the causes of diseases into three general types:

1. Internal
2. External
3. Others

Internal Causes of Illness

Its affirmed that the main internal causes of imbalance in the body are essentially psychological and are known as the six emotions:

1. Grief
2. Worry
3. Sadness
4. Fear
5. Frustration
6. Anger

In some cases we find strong evidence of some of these emotions while in other cases the difference is more a question of degrees, such as with sadness and suffering, fear and terror.

Taking the concept of the relationship between the five elements, the emotions are associated with the organic system in the following way:

EMOTION	ZANG	FU
Grief	Lungs	Large intestine
Worry	Spleen	Stomach
Sadness	Heart	Small intestine
Fear	Kidneys	Bladder
Frustration	Hormonal	Circulatory
Anger	Liver	Gall bladder

The feeling of emotion is intrinsic to the human experience and in Chinese medicine these emotions are as important in maintaining good health as they are relevant in the causation of disease.

It is always considered a question of degree. The six emotions are considered neither good nor bad; the important thing is that they remain in a balance. Below, different emotions are described and the way in which they can cause disharmony is also explained.

Anger

Anger includes all variety of associated emotions, such as resentment, irritability and frustration. Anger affects the liver and provokes a stagnation in the energy of the liver which can cause headaches, confusion and other symptoms. In the long run it can cause arterial hypertension and problems related to the stomach and spleen.

Happiness and Sadness

The idea of happiness refers to a state of agitation or over excitement more than an idea of profound well being.

The organ which is most directly affected is the heart. Excessive stimulation can cause fire/heat in the heart, which manifests itself in symptoms such as agitation, insomnia or palpitations. Sadness is the opposite feeling.

Sadness and suffering

Lungs are directly related to these emotions. A normal and healthy way of expressing sadness or suffering would be to cry, an act which comes from deep within the lungs, which brings about a deep breath and an expulsion of air. However, unresolved sadness can become chronic and create an imbalance in the lungs and weaken the *Chi* of the lungs, which interferes with their capacity to circulate energy.

Worry

In Chinese medicine, worry is considered as the result of excessive mental or intellectual stimulation.

The organ which is at utmost threat is the spleen. Insufficient amount of energy to the spleen can result in anxiety, restlessness and an inability to concentrate. The condition is further worsened in individuals who exhibit this kind of behavior as they generally have unhealthy and irregular eating habits, which makes the state of the spleen even worse.

Fear and terror

Fear is a normal human emotion which helps us to adapt to situations, but when it becomes chronic and the cause of the fear cannot be treated directly, it causes an imbalance. Kidneys are the most threatened organ. When the energy in the kidneys is exhausted, it provokes a shortage of yin, which in turn causes heat loss symptoms. For example, night time sweats or dryness in the mouth. A majority of people experience a gamut of emotions which varies in intensity. The important thing is how these emotions are dealt with; some people have more difficulty in dealing with them than others. It is important to take into account how these emotions influence the balance of energy in the body and in what shape or form these circumstances can cause an imbalance.

External Causes of Imbalance

Chinese medicine considers that there are six external causes of imbalance related to the climatic conditions. They are known under different names, the six pernicious influences, the six pathogenic factors or six bad externals:

1.   Cold
2.   Wind

3.   Humidity
4.   Fire or heat
5.   Dryness
6.   Heat of summer

Lifestyle factors

We are all conscious of the general stress of daily life and western medicine recognizes that these factors can have a big influence on our health and well being. Chinese medicine recognizes the importance of lifestyle in a similar way, although it is interpreted differently.

Work

The nature and quantity of work done by an individual has a profound influence on his energy system. An excess of physical work can damage the energy, with too much stimulation leading to atrophy the lungs. Too much mental activity harms the spleen and depletes the yin. A person who works outside is much more exposed to the cold, humidity, wind, heat, etc.

Exercise

The quantity and type of exercise that one does exerts an influence over him. In the same way, a lack of exercise can at times cause stagnation in energy. No specific exercise is bad or good in itself, but if taken in extremes can cause a noticeable imbalance.

Diet

The stomach and spleen are incharge of processing ingested food, which then passes to the lungs and this forms a fundamental part of the production of energy in the body. With regards to diet, the Chinese focus mainly on balance. If an individual follows a good balanced diet, the spleen stays healthy and the body will have sufficient energy.

Sexual activity

In Chinese medicine, sexual activity is considered very important, not just for the energy of the kidneys but for energy as a whole. It believes that insufficient sexual activity can cause problems in the general state of health of the individual.

It is clear that inner emotions as much as external influences are responsible for many different kinds of imbalances, which can manifest themselves as physical symptoms. Chinese medicine studies the way in which a combination of influences can conspire to create a picture of diseases within an individual.

WAYS OF DIAGNOSIS

In any process of evaluation it is vital to look at all the information. Without this appraisal/information it is impossible to formulate a hypothesis about the functions of the body and mind.

In Chinese medicine, the diagnostic process is developed from four perspectives, the four acknowledgements:

1. Visual examination
2. Auscultation and olfactory examination
3. History
4. Tactile exploration

When all of this information has been assembled from each of these four perspectives you have a complete picture.

THE TWELVE ORDINARY MERIDIANS

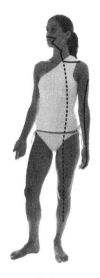

Colon

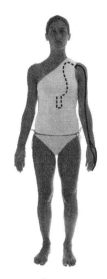

Lung

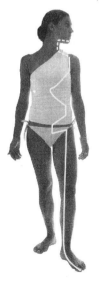

Spleen/Pancreas

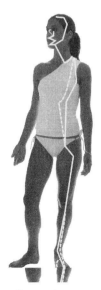

Stomach

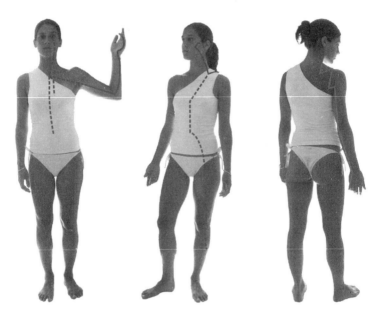

Heart   Small intestine

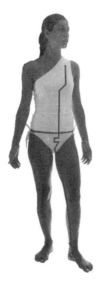

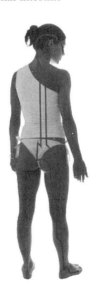

Kidney   Bladder

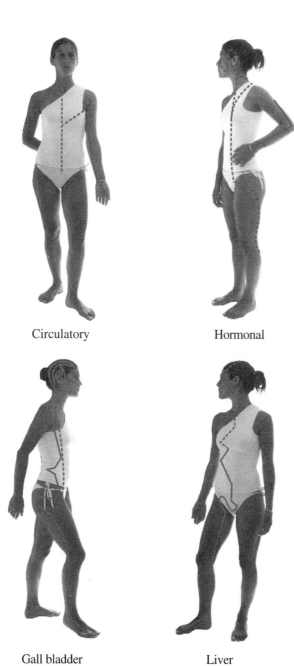

Circulatory   Hormonal

Gall bladder   Liver

TWO EXTRAORDINARY MERIDIANS

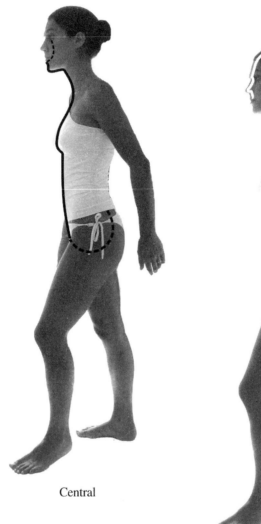

Central

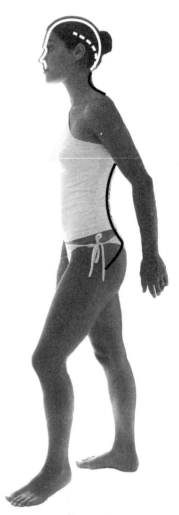

Governor

CHAPTER 8

The Fourteen Muscular Groups

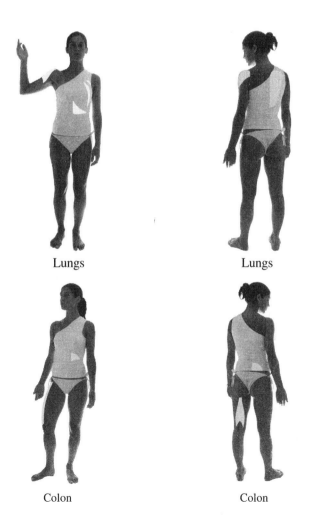

Lungs   Lungs

Colon   Colon

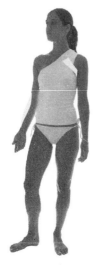

Stomach

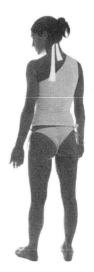

Stomach

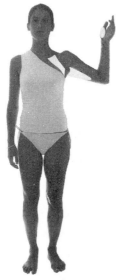

Spleen/Pancreas

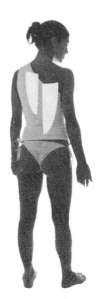

Spleen/Pancreas

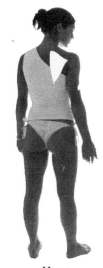

Heart

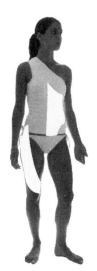

Small intestine

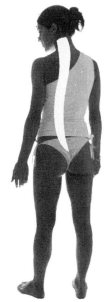

Bladder

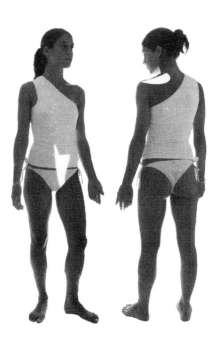

Kidney

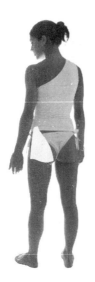 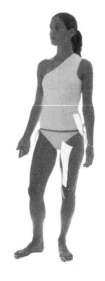

Circulatory

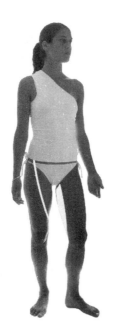 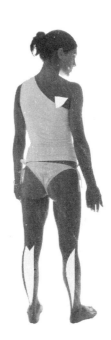

Hormonal

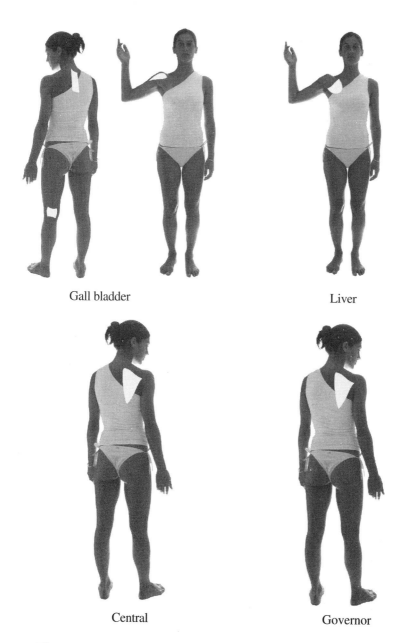

Gall bladder   Liver

Central   Governor

Illustration: The fourteen muscular groups related to meridians

Over a long period of time physicians have studied the effects of light or color stimulation. Doctors have used electromagnetic energies scientifically for treatment, diagnosis, radiographs, radiotherapy, infra-red, LASER therapy, etc. But long before, oriental cultures were using electrical energies to achieve an effect on the energy currents of the meridians, to treat a sick person using visible light/color, on the same vibration as the waves of the meridian energy flow.

The meridian colours used in Facial Reflexology concept are from an old school called "black hat school" that utilizes different colours of meridians from the claccic school of Chinese medicine. The "black hat school" is a synthesis of Chinese, Tibetan and Indian theories.

1.   Lung and Large intestine – Blue

2.   Spleen and Stomach – Yellow

3.   Heart and Small intestine – Violet

4.   Kidneys and Bladder – Red

5.   Endocrine and Circulation – Orange

6.   Liver and Gall bladder – Green

The colors are also used for analysis:

1.   The color of the skin – For lungs and colon

2.   The color of the lips – For spleen and stomach

3.   The color of the tongue – For heart and small intestine

4.   The color of the arms – For kidneys and bladder.

5.   The color of the complexion – For endocrine and circulation.

6.   The color of the nails and eyes (the white part) – For liver and gall bladder

Acupuncture is a customary innocuous procedure, free from side effects and something which as a rule, can provide relief, and improve many health problems, diseases and illnesses, syndromes and symptoms. It is economic and easily applied by trained professionals: medical personnel, nurses, anesthetists or physiotherapists and other professionals working in the health sector.

The main indications of acupuncture are diseases that cause pain. For this reason the most important part of the procedure is the analysis. It is also effective in a majority of psychosomatic problems, which are so common nowadays.

In the inter-regional seminar of the World Health Organization in Beijing in 1979, acupuncture was recommended to treat a group of illnesses and diseases based mainly on clinical experience and not necessarily controlled clinical research. The majority of participants were medical personnel from the west, as opposed to traditional Chinese medicine. The diseases and problems were:

Respiratory: Acute sinusitis, acute rhinitis, nasal catarrh, acute tonsillitis, acute bronchitis, bronchial asthma (mainly in children and complicated cases).

Gastro-intestinal: Spasms of the esophagus and cardiac end of stomach, acute and chronic gastritis, gastric hyperacidity, gastroptosis, chronic duodenal ulcers (analgesia) acute duodenal ulcer (without complications), acute and chronic colitis, acute basillary dysentery (Japanese dysentery), constipation, diarrhea, adynamic ileus.

Eyes: Acute conjuctivitis, central retinitis, myopia in children, cataract.

Mouth: Toothache, post-extraction pain in tooth and gingivitis.

Neurological Problem: Headache, migraine, trigeminal neuralgia, facial paralysis, peripheral neuropathies, sequele of poliomyelitis, Meniere's disease, neurogenic bladder, nocturnal enuresis, intercostal neuralgia, cervicobrachial syndrome, paresthesias, frozen shoulder, tennis elbow, sciatica, lumbo-sacral pain and osteoarthritis.

CHAPTER 9

Meridianology

COLON/LUNG MERIDIAN

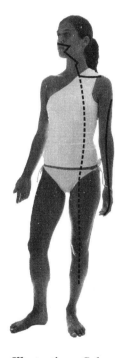

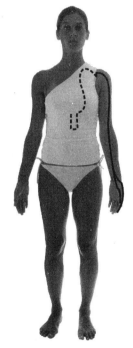

Illustration: *Colon meridian*

Illustration: *Lung meridian*

The main meridian of the colon begins at the tip of the index finger, it goes up to the outside of the arm, along the back of the shoulder and in to the corner of the lips and ends under the nose.

The main meridian of the lungs begins in the trunk and goes to the underarm area, down at the inside of the arm and ends at the tip of the thumb.

LUNG MERIDIAN

Lung has no NP point.

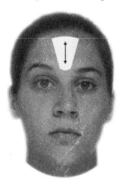

Indian Zone

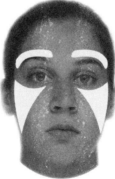

Oriental Zone

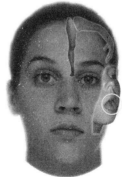

Oriental zone for the sensory organs

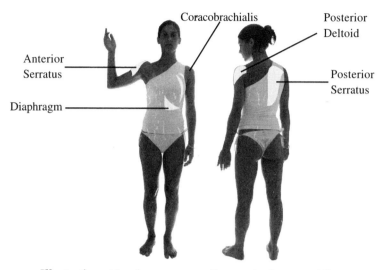

Illustration: Muscles corresponding to the lung meridian

Sensitive organs: Nose   *Tissue:* Skin and body hair
Sense: Smell   *Liquid:* Mucus secretion
Taste: Spicy   *Made worse by:* Lying down
Color: Blue   *Season:* Autumn

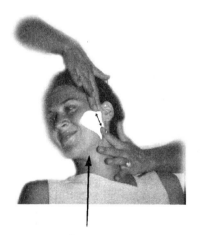

Lung zone
Illustration: Lung zone on left side

Lung zone

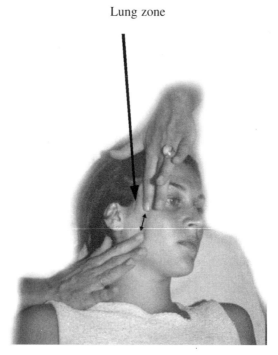

Illustration: Lung zone on right side

Lungs are responsible for respiration. Inhalation is the process by which we get the necessary oxygen to live and exhalation means expulsion of the air mixed with carbon dioxide. The respiratory passages include nose, pharynx, larynx, trachea, bronchi and bronchioles. Air is inhaled and passed through the nasal passages where it is filtered, heated and humidified. The process continues as the air goes through the pharynx, larynx, trachea and bronchia to the lungs.

The bronchioles end in the alveoli (tiny air sacs in the lungs), where the exchange of gases between oxygen and carbon dioxide takes place.

COLON MERIDIAN

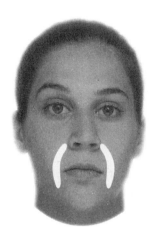

Indian zone

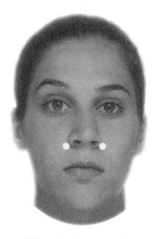

NP point for the colon

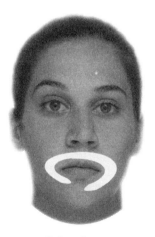

Oriental zone

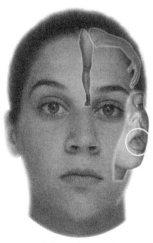

Oriental zone for the
sensory organs

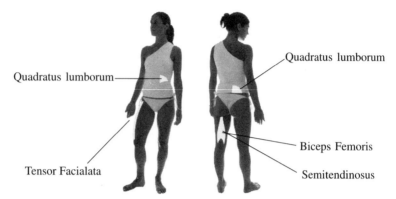

Illustration: Muscles corresponding to the colon meridian

The colon meridian acts upon the same sensory organs, tissues, etc. and produces the same symptoms as the lung meridian. **It shares the same personality traits and emotional status as the lung:** weeping, negativity and fear of loss.

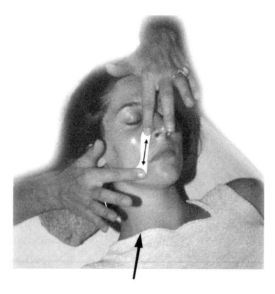

Colon zone

Illustration: Colon zone of right side

Colon zone

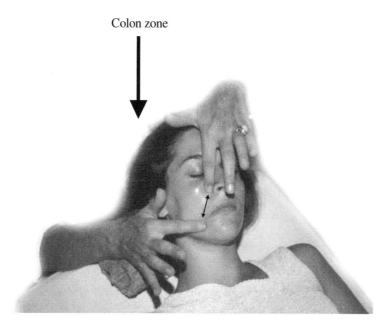

Illustration: *Colon zone of left side*

The large intestine is made up of the blind gut, the colon and the rectum. The blind gut is a short section shaped like a sack in which a small protuberance called the appendix is found, their function is to prepare cells to defend the organism.

The colon ascends vertically, passing below the stomach and descending as far as the rectum. Rectum is the last part of the digestive tube which ends in the anus. The main function of the large intestine is to absorb salts, minerals and water and make feces – food which has not been absorbed by the small intestine but instead, fermented by bacteria in the large intestine.

THE STOMACH/SPLEEN-PANCREAS MERIDIAN

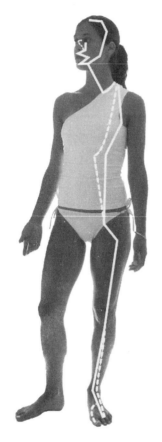

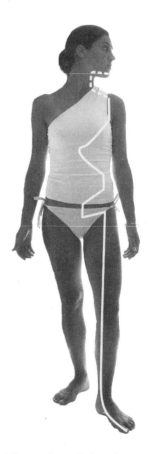

Illustration: *Stomach meridian*

The main meridian of the stomach starts underneath the eye and follows the line of the jaw bone as far as the ear, goes above the eyebrows, down the neck towards the thorax and stomach, down the middle of the leg, ending in the second toe.

Illustration: *Spleen/pancreas meridian*

The main meridian of the spleen/pancreas starts in the large toe, in the inside of the leg and goes up towards the chest as far as the collar bone.

STOMACH MERIDIAN

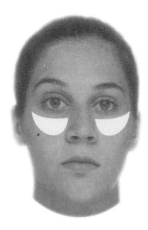

Indian zone

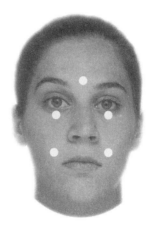

NP point for the stomach

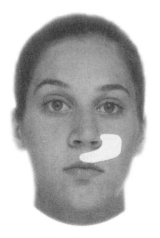

Oriental zone

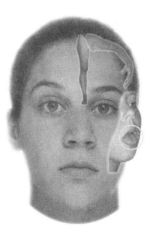

Oriental zone for the
sensory organs

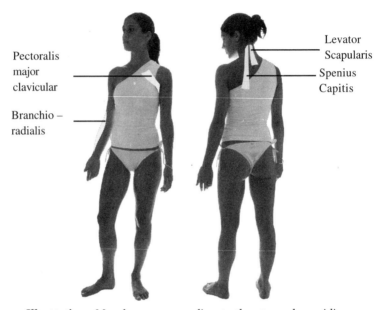

Pectoralis
major
clavicular

Branchio –
radialis

Levator
Scapularis

Spenius
Capitis

Illustration: Muscles corresponding to the stomach meridian

Sensitive organs: Mouth and lips   *Tissue:* Connective tissue
Sense: Taste   *Liquid:* Saliva and lymph
Taste: Sweet   *Made worse by:* Sitting
Color: Yellow   *Season:* Last Summer
                                  (canicula)

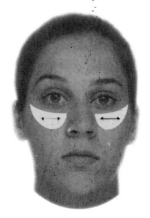

Stomach zone

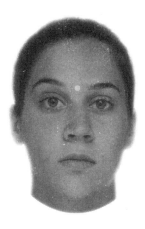

Illustration: *Extra acupuncture point for the stomach*

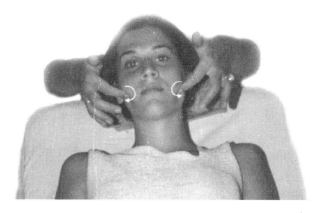

Illustration: *Acupuncture point for the stomach*

Before the food and nutrients reach the *stomach*, they go through a process of conversion, which begins in the mouth when the food is mixed with saliva. The result is a substance known as bolus, which then goes to the digestive tube, towards the stomach where it is transformed into chyme with help from the digestive juices. The pylorus and cardia are valves that open and close the stomach.

SPLEEN/PANCREAS MERIDIAN

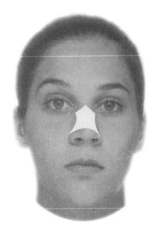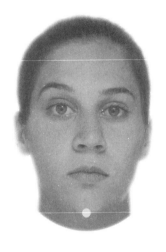

Indian zone

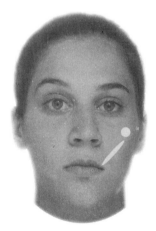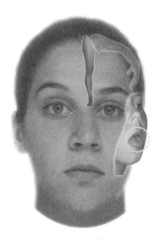

Oriental zone   Oriental zone for the
                                        sensory organs

Illustration: The spleen and the pancreas are stimulated at
the same time

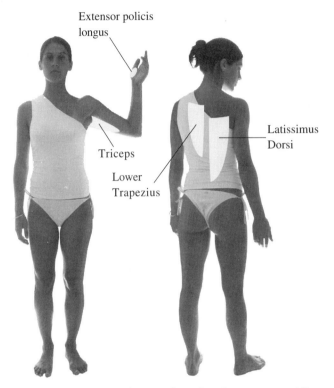

Illustration: *Muscles corresponding to the spleen/pancreas meridian*

The meridian for the spleen/pancreas acts upon the same sensory organs, tissues etc. and produces the same symptoms as the stomach meridian. **It shares the same personality traits and emotional status as the stomach:** sadness, crying, negativity, stress and shock.

SMALL INTESTINE/HEART MERIDIAN

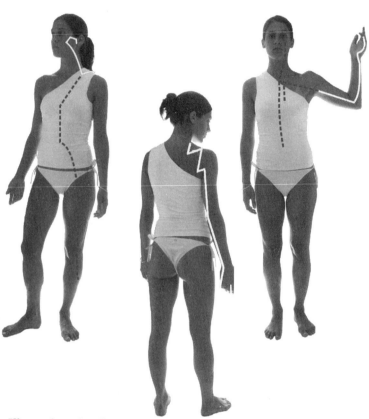

Illustration: *Small intestine meridian*

Illustration: *Heart meridian*

The main meridian of the small intestine starts on the outer point of the little finger and goes up underneath the arm, behind the shoulder to the neck and cheek bones and finishes near the ear.

The main meridian of the heart starts in the arm pit, goes down and inside of the arm and ends at the tip of the little finger.

HEART MERIDIAN

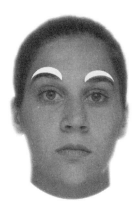

Indian zone

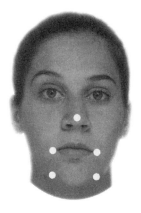

NP point for the heart

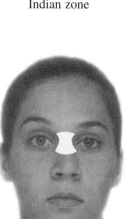

Oriental zone

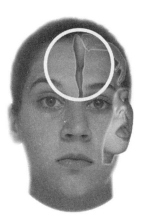

Oriental zone for
the sensory organs

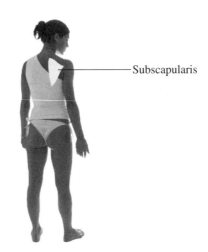

——— Subscapularis

Illustration: *Muscles corresponding to the heart meridian*

Sensitive organs: Tongue   *Tissue:* Brain, veins
Sense: Taste   *Liquid:* Perspiration
Taste: Bitter   *Made worse by:* Walking
Color: Violet   *Season:* Summer

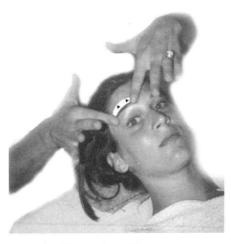

Illustration: *Heart zone*

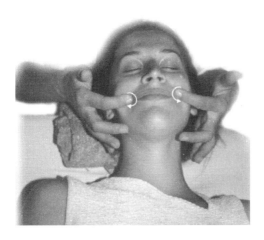

Illustration: Extra neurovascular points for the heart

The heart is incharge of pumping the blood across the body. It is divided into two halves, the right side and the left side and is separated by a thin wall, which prevents any type of communication; each half is divided again into two parts – the auricular and the ventricular. The blood circulates via blood vessels across the body.

There are three different types of blood vessels:

1. The arteries circulate the blood that comes from the heart.
2. The veins carry the blood from the tissues to the auricular part of the heart.
3. The capillaries, which are very fine blood vessels, found inside all tissues.

SMALL INTESTINE MERIDIAN

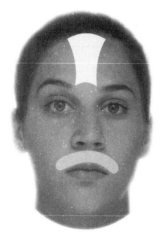

Indian zone

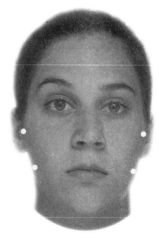

NP point for the small
intestine

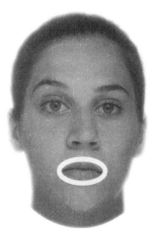

Oriental zone for the
small intestine

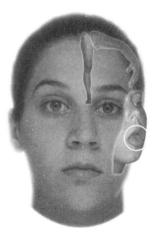

Oriental zone for the
sensory organs

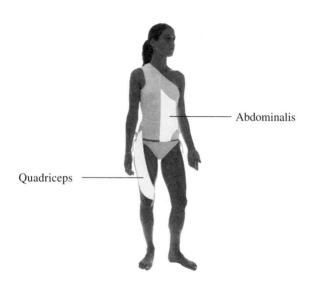

Illustration: Muscles corresponding to the small intestine meridian

The small intestine meridian acts upon the same sensory organs and tissues, and produces the same symptoms as the heart meridian. **It shares the same personality traits and emotional status with the heart meridian:** constant talking, nervous movements, hysterical laughter.

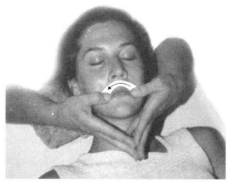

Illustration: Small intestine zone

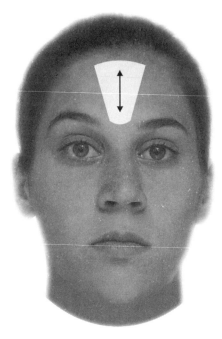

Illustration: *Small intestine zone*

The small intestine is filled with chyle, this is due to the digestion process carried out by the intestinal juices, pancreatic juices and bile. Once the food is changed into nutrients, intestinal absorption is carried out. This consists of passing the nutrients through the walls of the intestine to the blood vessels which distribute the nutrients to all the tissues of body. The small intestine is a tube, which is seven meters long and divided into three sections: duodenum, jejunum and ileum.

KIDNEY/BLADDER MERIDIAN

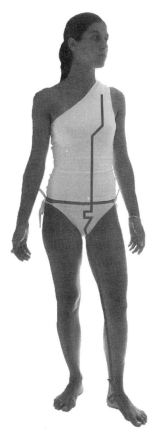

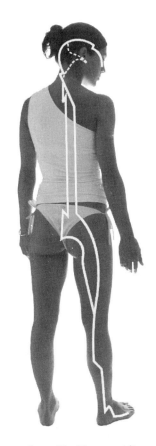

Illustration: Kidney meridian

Illustration: Bladder meridian

The main meridian of the kidney begins in the sole of the foot, makes a loop when it reaches the ankle, then goes up through the leg along the sexual organs, up to the stomach and ends at the collar bone.

The main meridian of the bladder begins in the inner side of the eye, passes over the top of the head, down the neck where it splits in two and runs parallel down the back, buttocks, hamstrings. It rejoins behind the knee and ends at the tip of the little toe.

KIDNEY MERIDIAN

The kidneys don't have NP points

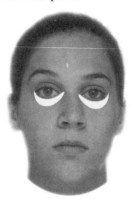

South American Indian zone

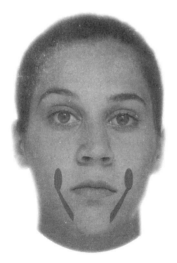

Oriental zone

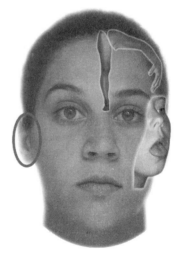

Zone for the sensory organs

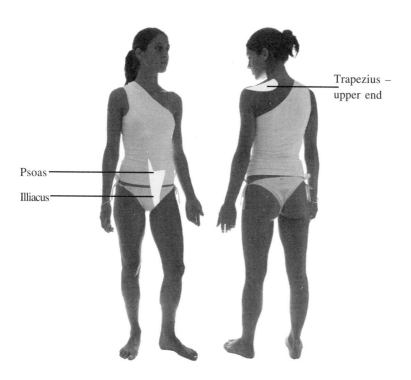

Illustration: *Muscles corresponding to the kidney meridian*

Sensitive organs: Ear   *Tissue:* Bones, nails, teeth, hair.
Sense: Hearing   *Liquid:* Urine
Taste: Salty   *Made worse by:* Standing still
Color: Red   *Season:* Winter

The kidneys and urinary passages make up part of the excretory system. The kidneys are bean shaped organs, 2 in number and situated in the lumbar region, on either side of the spine. Kidneys are formed by nephrons which are its structural and functional unit. The urinary passages carry the urine from the kidneys to the urethra.

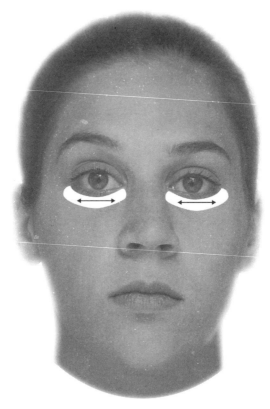

Illustration: South American Indian zone

Excretion consists of elimination of waste products from the blood. Waste products are also eliminated through the sweat glands in the skin. They have a globular part that filters blood and a duct that goes through the different layers of skin and reaches the surface. Both, urine and sweat are largely made up of water, mineral salts, urea and uric acid. Sweat is more diluted than urine and has a double function – elimination of wastes and to regulate body temperature.

BLADDER MERIDIAN

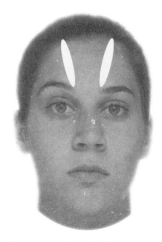

South American Indian zone

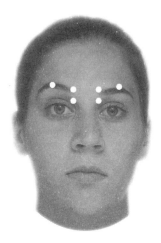

Neurovascular NP point

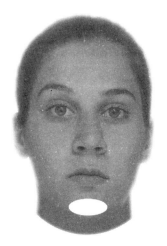

Oriental zone

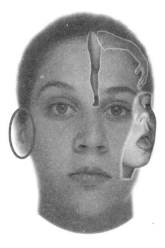

Oriental zone for the
sensory organs

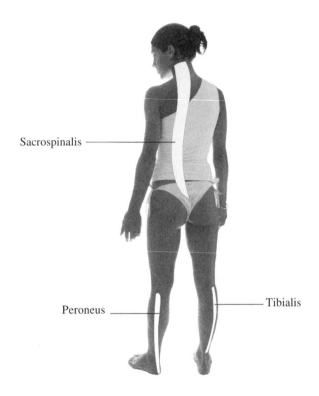

Sacrospinalis

Peroneus

Tibialis

Illustration: Muscles corresponding to the bladder meridian

The bladder meridian acts upon the same sensory organs, tissues, etc. and produces the same symptoms as the kidney meridian. **It shares the same personality traits and emotional status as the kidney:** passivity, fear, terror.

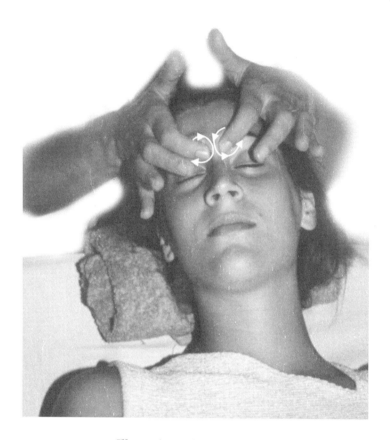

Illustration: *The bladder zone*

The bladder: The urine collects in the renal pelvis before sliding gently into the urethra towards the bladder. When the bladder is full, impulses are sent to the brain giving the information that the bladder needs to be evacuated. The muscles of the bladder then relax, the urethra opens and the walls of the bladder contract allowing the urine to be excreted from the body.

HORMONAL / CIRCULATION MERIDIAN

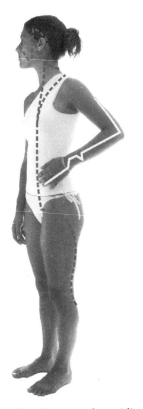
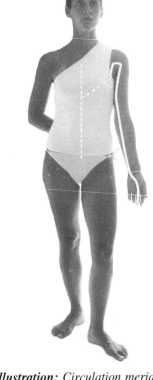

Illustration: Hormonal meridian   *Illustration: Circulation meridian*

The main meridian of the hormonal system begins on the tip of the ring finger. It passes up the back of the hand between the ring and little finger. It goes up the side of the neck to split in 2 branches on either side of the ear. 1 branch arrives at the temple and ends at a part outside the eyebrows and the other branch stops at the top of the ear.

The main circulation meridian begins near the nipple. Then goes across the chest, down the inner side of the arm to the palm of the hand and ends on the tip of the middle finger.

HORMONAL MERIDIAN

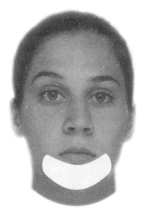

Zone for the hormonal
system

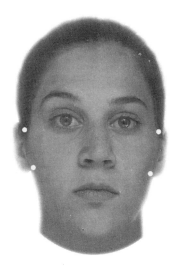

NP point

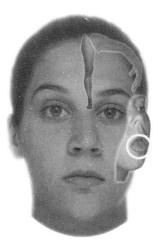

Zone for the sensory
organs

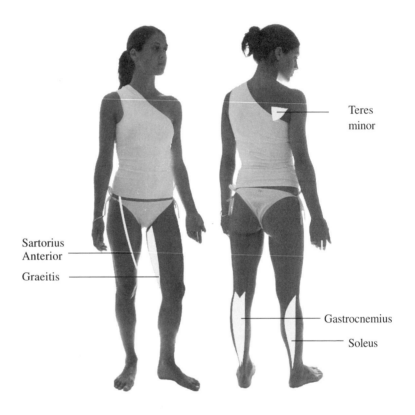

Teres
minor

Sartorius
Anterior

Graeitis

Gastrocnemius

Soleus

Illustration: Muscles corresponding to the endocrine meridian

Sensitive organs: Tongue
Sense: Taste
Taste: Bitter
Color: Orange

Tissue: Brain, nervous system,
     capillaries.
Liquid: Perspiration
Made worse by: Walking
Season: Summer

The hormonal system regulates different parts of the body by means of chemical messages or hormones, produced by cells grouped in the endocrine glands. The feedback mechanism controls hormone production; if there is sufficient concentration of a certain hormone in the blood, the feedback mechanism will curb its production. Similarly, if there is insufficient concentration, it will promote the release of the necessary hormone.

The endocrine glands are: pituitary gland, thyroid glands, the parathyroid glands, adrenal glands and the pancreas.

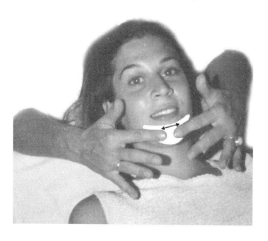

Illustration: Hormonal Zone

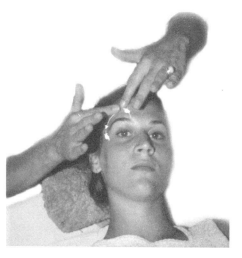

Illustration: Zone for the cortex of the brain

CIRCULATORY MERIDIAN

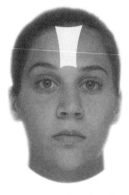

There is no NP point
for the circulation

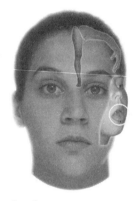

Zone for the circulation   Zone for the sensory organs
(shared also by the small intestine)

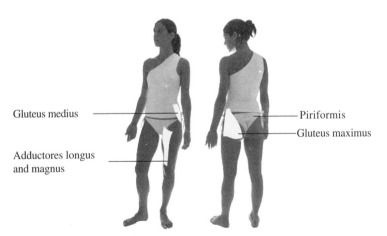

Gluteus medius   Piriformis
                                                                  Gluteus maximus

Adductores longus
and magnus

Illustration: *Muscles corresponding to the circulation meridian*

The circulation meridian acts upon the same sensory organs, tissues, etc. and produces the same symptoms as the endocrine meridian.

It shares the same personality traits and emotional status as the endocrine meridian: hysteria, frustration, restlessness and excessive verbosity.

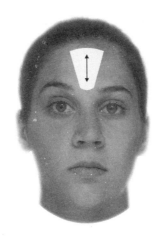

Illustration: *Circulation zone*

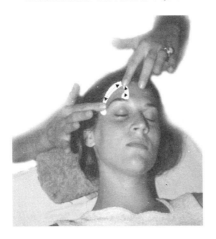

Illustration: *Zone for the sensory organs*

The circulatory system: There are two types of liquid in the body – blood and lymph, both of which flows separately. Oxygen and nutrients are circulated across the body through blood, where as carbon dioxide and other waste products are collected from the body. The lymphatic circulation is incharge of collecting existing liquids between the cells and carrying, fats which are absorbed in the intestine.

LIVER / GALL BLADDER MERIDIAN

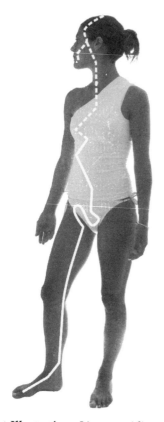

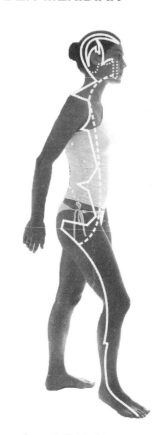

Illustration: Liver meridian   *Illustration:* Gall bladder meridian

The main meridian of the liver begins in the center of the big toe beneath the nail, passes between this and the next toe, going up the inside leg and thigh near the sex organs, then towards the waist, and ends near the nipple.

The main meridian of the gall bladder starts in the outermost point of the eye and moves up towards the center of the forehead, goes down to the neck, the shoulders, front of the thorax and abdomen, to the hip bone, moving down the outside of the leg, finishing at the fourth toe.

LIVER MERIDIAN

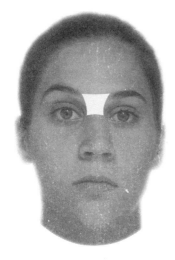

South American Indian Zone

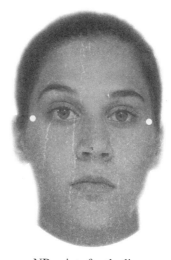

NP points for the liver

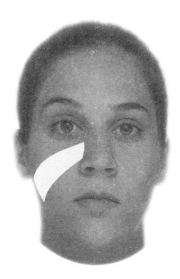

Oriental Zone

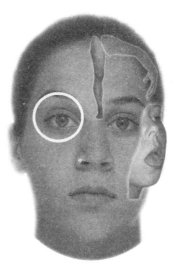

Zone for the sensory organs

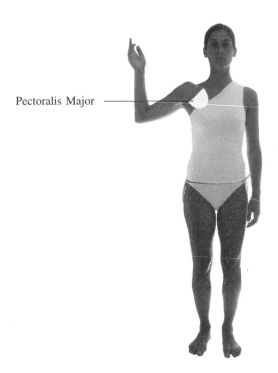

Pectoralis Major

Illustration: Muscles corresponding to the liver meridian

Sensitive organs: Eye   *Tissue:* Muscles and tendons
Sense: Sight   *Liquid:* Tears
Taste: Acidic   *Made worse by:* Excessive visual use
Color: Green   *Season:* Spring

The liver is a gland weighing about 2 kg and is responsible for making bile, a liquid which is stored in the gall bladder and helps in the digestion of fat.

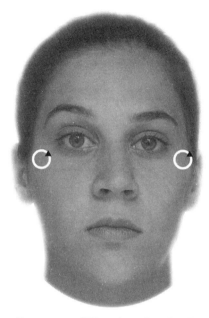

Illustration: NP points for the liver

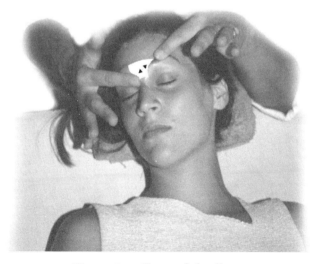

Illustration: Zone of the liver

GALL BLADDER MERIDIAN

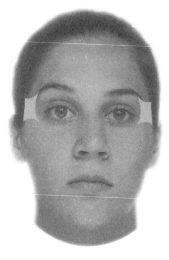

South American Indian zone

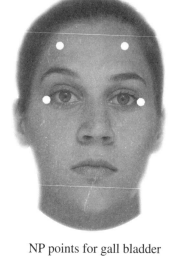

NP points for gall bladder

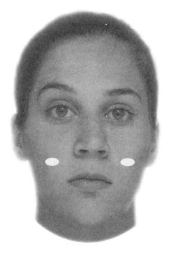

Oriental zone

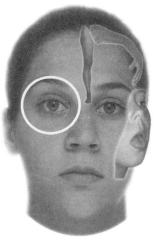

Oriental zone for the
sensory organs

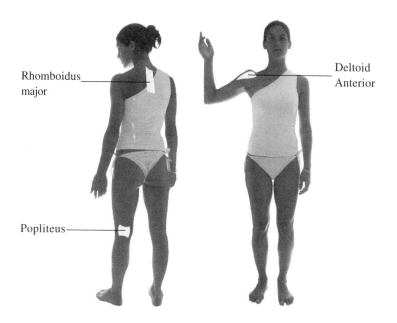

Rhomboidus major

Deltoid Anterior

Popliteus

Illustration: Muscles corresponding to the gall bladder meridian

The gall bladder meridian acts upon the same sensory organs, tissues, etc. and produces the same symptoms as the liver meridian. **It shares a similar personality traits and emotional status as the liver:** aggression, arrogance, irritability, strength of character, jealousy and loud-mouthed behavior.

Bile is stored in the gall bladder and released when there is food in the small intestine. It also has other functions such as storing and transformation of nutrients and the cleansing of organism – essential, since the liver stores potentially toxic substances such as medicines, additives, etc.

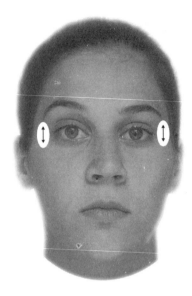

Illustration: *Gall bladder zone*

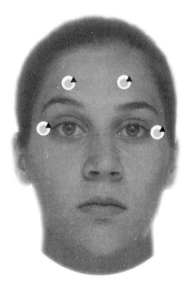

Illustration: *NP points for the gall bladder*

CENTRAL / GOVERNOR MERIDIAN

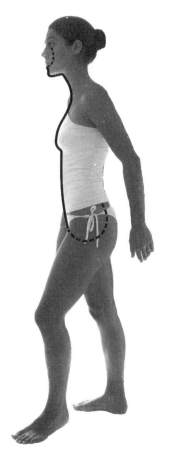 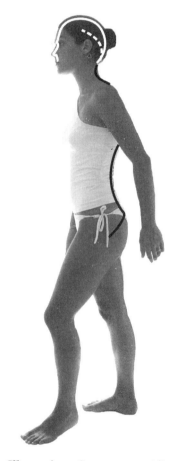

Illustration: *Central meridian*

Illustration: *Governor meridian*

The central meridian begins at the top of the pelvis and ends below the mouth.

The main governor meridian starts in the coccyx and ends above the mouth.

THE GOVERNOR MERIDIAN

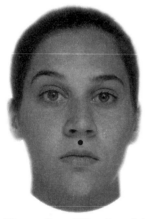

Illustration: NP point of the
Governor meridian

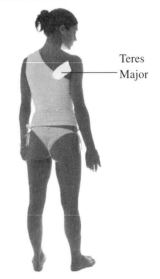

Teres
Major

Illustration: Muscle corresponding
to Governor meridian

The governor and central meridian are not related to any vital organ but are responsible for maintaining the balance of the electric current between the twelve meridians. Stimulating the neurovascular point of the governor, helps the following problems:

1. Illnesses of the mouth, herpes and ulcers
2. Infections
3. Any weakness of the immune system
4. Spinal problems
5. Illnesses of the anus and rectum
6. Balance problems and mental illnesses
7. Deafness and dumbness
8. Epilepsy
9. Infantile fits
10. Muscular cramps

CENTRAL AND GOVERNOR MERIDIAN

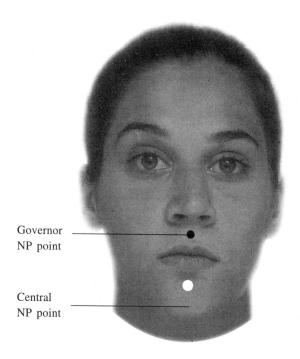

Governor
NP point

Central
NP point

Illustration: NP point of the governor and central meridian

The nervous system is made up of the central nervous system, the peripheral nervous system and the autonomous nervous system or vegetative (sympathetic and parasympathetic) nervous system.

1. They detect stimuli in the environment – receptors.
2. They drive sensory information – sensory system.
3. They process information and issue commands – central nervous system.
4. They drive the orders – motor system.
5. They carry out a motor and secretory job – effectors.

CENTRAL MERIDIAN (REN)

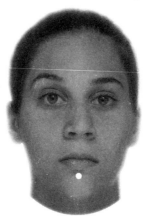

Illustration: NP point for the central meridian

The NP point of the central meridian helps in following problems:

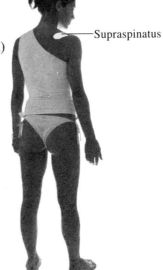

1. Facial paralysis
2. Excessive salivation
3. Speech problems (Dysphonia)
4. Heart problems
5. Lung illnesses
6. Stomach problems
7. Intestinal dysfunction
8. Uro-genital problems

Supraspinatus

Illustration: Muscle corresponding to central meridian

The Interconnections of the Meridians

The electric current between the meridians is never interrupted. It begins in the lung meridian and passes through all the meridians until it arrives in the liver, where it returns and begins its route again in the lung meridian.

This large electric system is divided into three smaller systems, each containing four meridians, a pair of meridians and the interrelated meridians:

1. The frontal meridian system: lung, colon, stomach, spleen.
2. The posterior meridian system: heart, small intestine, bladder and kidneys.
3. The lateral meridian system: blood circulation, hormonal system, liver and gall bladder.

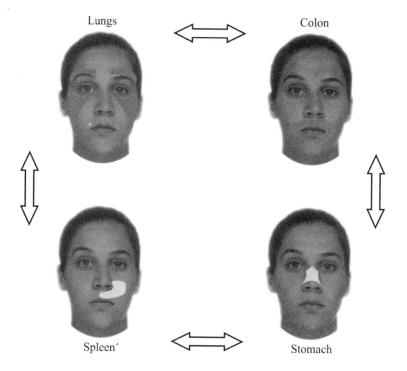

Lungs   Colon

Spleen'   Stomach

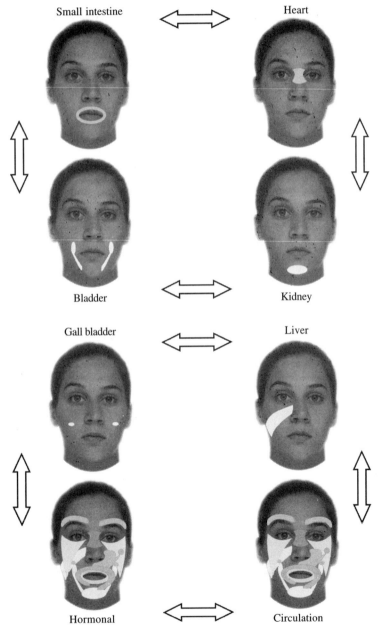

Illustration: *The pairs of meridians and their interconnections*

CHAPTER 10

Physical and Mental Map of the Body

THE 'PHYSICAL BODY'

The concept of cibernetics include treating the 'physical body', this is done through a map of the physical body on the face.

The stimulation technique has been developed from studies conducted on the nose in facial acupuncture and the results were impressive because it works upon the central nervous system and the muscular skeletal system.

With a patient lying down, the therapist sits behind him/her and from this angle studies the face. In some cases it is possible to see certain deviations in the face. These deviations are shown in the rest of the body. Thus, not only is it possible to observe postural problems in the body by studying the face but one can help treat them simply by means of facial stimulation.

Bad posture always affects spinal nerves, which means that the impulse cannot flow freely through the organs and muscles. This can cause problems at a chemical, organic and hormonal level. A decrease in the impulses in the spinal nerves can also cause mental and psychological problems.

The stimulation is carried out by applying pressure with the fingertips throughout the zones that represent the physical body. Starting with the zone representing the face and working downwards, stimulating the zones of the arms, hands, spinal column, and lastly the legs and feet.

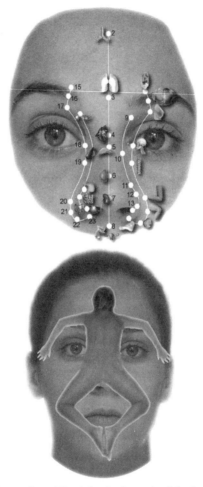

Illustration: *The 'physical map' of the body*

The treatment ends with a stimulation known as balancing, which involves finding which ever plexus zone has the most deposits, choosing the corresponding neurovascular acupuncture point and applying pressure to these points (illustration, page 115).

It is recommended that this part of the treatment be done after the six basic steps have been completed.

PLEXUS BALANCING

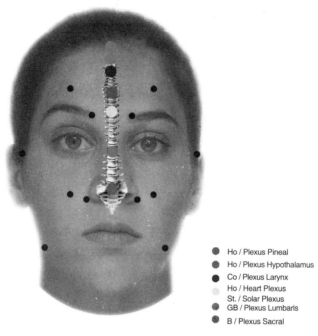

Ho / Plexus Pineal
Ho / Plexus Hypothalamus
Co / Plexus Larynx
Ho / Heart Plexus
St. / Solar Plexus
GB / Plexus Lumbaris
B / Plexus Sacral

Illustration: *Plexus balancing*

Press on both points which belong to the plexus corresponding to the hormonal gland and the point corresponding to the meridian (NP point) with the biggest deposit and hold for one minute.

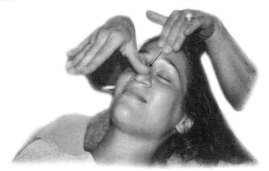

The movement works upon the circuit mentioned below:

Gland	Meridian	Vertebrae	Plexus	Emotion
Pineal, Pituitary Hypothalamus	Hormonal/ Circulation	1-5 C	Pineal/ Thalamus (1-2)	Guilt, loss of identity
Thyroid, Parathyroid	Colon/ Lung	7 C 1-2-3, 12-T	Larynx (3)	Dominance
Thymus	Heart/ Small intestine	2-3, 8-11 T, 5-L	Heart (4)	Frustration, personality disorder
Pancreas	Stomach/ Spleen	2-7 C 3-8 T	Solar (5)	Nervousness
Adrenals	Liver/ Gall bladder	3-4-5-6 T	Lumbar (6)	Feeling of being inferior
Reproductive glands	Kidneys/ Bladder	9-10-11 T 1-2, 5 L	Sacral (7)	Fear, loss of control

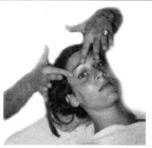
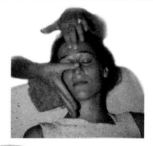
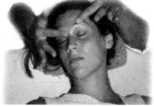

THE PSYCHOLOGICAL MAP

The other cibernetic map is the 'psychological map.' This is carried out by working simultaneously with both hands:

1. The hands move in a circular direction over the forehead, with each hand working on one side of the forehead.
2. Followed by working the area's for the hand.
3. Lastly ending on the area's for the feet, continuing to work on each side of the face at the same time.

These movements have a powerful effect upon the coordination of the two hemispheres of the brain.

In the basic treatment that is, the seven steps, the 'psychological Map' is always the last to be stimulated.

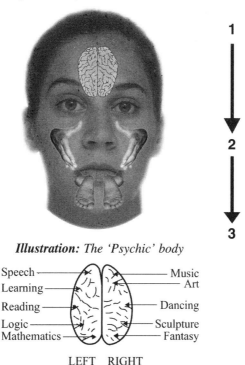

Illustration: *The 'Psychic' body*

Speech — Music
Learning — Art
Reading — Dancing
Logic — Sculpture
Mathematics — Fantasy

LEFT   RIGHT

CHAPTER 11

The Five Elements Theory

THE FIVE ELEMENTS THEORY

The origins of Chinese philosophical thinking has its roots in **Taoism**. Basically, Taoism is largely based on observing nature and how it works. Chinese medicine gives rise to a metaphorical vision of the human body based on the observation of the exchanges of yin and yang in the natural world. The Chinese realized that there is an exchange of energy in everything. A seed (yin) becomes a plant (yang) which in turn returns to the earth (yin) to die. The same happens with the changes of season. Winter (yin) changes into summer (yang) during spring and summer changes into winter through autumn. It is not strange that the Chinese medical system frequently uses metaphors from the natural world. This idea is taken further in the five elements theory (also known as the five phases).

The five elements theory comes from observing the different groups of energetic processes, functions and characteristics of the natural world. The five elements with their properties are:

1. **Water:** Humid, cold, descent, fluid complacent.
2. **Fire:** Dry, heat and essential movement.
3. **Wood:** Growth, flexible and taking root strength.
4. **Metal:** Capacity to cut and lasting conduction.
5. **Earth:** Productive, fertile and potential for growth.

These characteristics are examples of how the elements can be understood, but the most important idea is that everything contains both yin and yang, which reflects the principle of duality and mutual interaction, which is a basic in Chinese thinking. They believe that each element has a series of connections as much in the natural world as in the human body.

Chinese medicine uses a system of interconnections between the five elements as a way of understanding how they support each other and control the different processes of the body. These interconnections are defined as cycles of Sheng and Ki.

The elements of the natural world are controlled amongst themselves as part of the process of balancing energy.

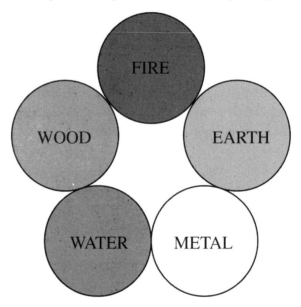

Illustration: 5 Elements in nature

For example, fire controls metal since it can melt it. In the same way water controls fire because it is capable of extinguishing it. In terms of Chinese medicine, the idea of control is understood as the part of the process by which one organ helps another. For example, lungs help to control the energy in the liver and thus, plays a part in making sure that it functions properly. An imbalance can be a consequence of a weakness in an organ and so the corresponding organ can give it the necessary support.

If the energy in the lungs is weak, the energy in the liver will have a tendency to be out of control and to increase disproportionately, which can manifest itself in the appearance of various problems such as headaches or arterial hypertension.

Problems can also appear in the opposite direction, which in this case would be interpreted as a revolt against the naturally controlling function. For example, if the spleen is too humid the balance can be broken and so the ability of the liver to move the energy around the body is diminished.

The system of the five elements is important in demonstrating the way in which Chinese medicine portions the Taoist idea of balance, the process and harmony in the natural world. In facial reflexology, the problems of the patients are seen from the perspective of the five elements theory and the intervention is based on said principles.

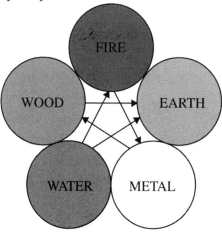

Illustration: *Control of elements; process of balancing energy*

CHAPTER 12

Cranial Acupressure

CRANIAL LINES AND POINTS

Cranial acupressure is based on the stimulation of different lines and points of the cranium, which stimulate the cerebral cortex. These points and lines which are related to the meridians and plexus have a direct connection to different organs and to the organic workings of the body too.

It is possible to monitor the function of the areas of the brain with different electronic devices, which tracks the functioning of brain; for example, the FXS machine that is used to diagnose brain effusions and clots and to check which bodily functions have stopped receiving nerve stimuli. Through stimulation of facial points and zones, it is possible in the same way to monitor if there are some changes in the function of the brain.

Oriental philosophy states that it is possible to send orders from the brain to different parts of the body and vice versa. It has been proven by experience that in situations such as paralysis, reduction in mobility, sensory confusion, etc. It is possible to speed up or to shorten the recuperation time if the cranial lines and points are stimulated.

The lines are stimulated simply by rubbing on both sides of the scalp simultaneously. The movement is similar to the movement used in ironing. It is done with the fingers and should last for 2 or 3 minutes per line, the pressure being firm but light. When stimulating by rubbing on the scalp it is important to work inside the corresponding brain area, but not necessarily to stimulate as puntual as when using needles.

The cranial points are then stimulated on both sides of the cranium simultaneously, using a light pressure lasting for about a minute.

Music therapy is recommended as an additional treatment for cranial therapy, especially for different types of learning and comprehending difficulties.

1. MOTOR LINE: Paralysis, reduction in mobility (phonetic line 1). The opposite side is stimulated – Heart point/line.

2. SENSORY LINE: Distributed to the face and extremities. Numbness and sensory confusion – Small intestine point/line.

3. VASOMOTOR: Edema, arterial hypertension – Spleen/ Pancreas point/line.

4. MOTOR AND FOOT SENSITIVITY: Sensory confusion, trembling in the calves – Small intestine point/line.

5. TREMOR LINE: Uncontrollable trembling, Parkinson's disease – Stomach point/line.

6. AUDITORY LINE: All types of auditory confusion – Kidney point/line.

7. PHONETIC LINE (III): Phonetic confusion – Lung point/ line.

8. PHONETIC LINE (II): Parietal tubercle – Phonetic confusion hormonal point.

9. VISUAL LINE: Blindness – Circulation point/line.

10. BALANCE LINE: Imbalance – Bladder point/line.

11. MIDDLE LINE: (Governor) – Heart point/line.

Cranial Lines

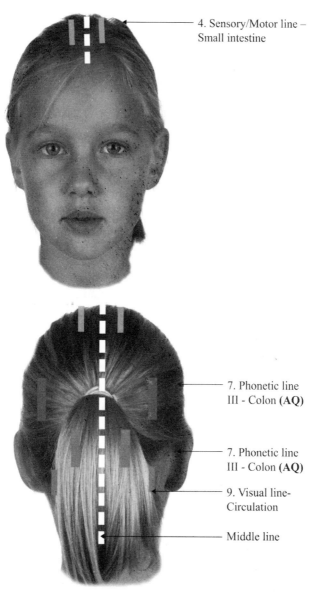

4. Sensory/Motor line –
Small intestine

7. Phonetic line
III - Colon **(AQ)**

7. Phonetic line
III - Colon **(AQ)**

9. Visual line-
Circulation

Middle line

Middle line

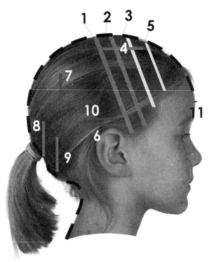

Illustration: *Cranial Lines*

1. MOTOR LINE: Paralysis, reduction in mobility (phonetic line 1) – Heart points/lines – 3

2. SENSORY LINE: To the face and extremities. Numbers and sensory confusion – Small intestine points/lines.

3. VASOMOTOR: Edema, arterial hypertension – Spleen/pancreas points/lines – 2

4. MOTOR AND FOOT SENSITIVITY: Sensory confusion, trembling in the calves – Small intestine points/lines – 4

5. TREMOR LINE: Uncontrollable trembling, Parkinson's disease – Stomach points/lines – 1

6. AUDITORY LINE: All types of auditory confusion – Kidney points/lines – 6

7. PHONETIC LINE (III) Phonetic confusion – Lung points/lines – 11

8. PHONETIC LINE (II): Parietal tubercle. Phonetic confusion – Hormonal points/lines – 8

9. VISUAL LINE: Blindness – Circulation points/lines – 7

10. BALANCE LINE: Imbalance – Bladder points/lines – 5

Illustration: *Cranial points which have a direct connection to the brain centers and to all the muscles of the body. The cranial points have a pulse which is dependent upon the lymphatic system. The points are stimulated by applying a gentle but firm pressure.*

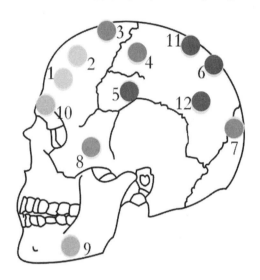

1. Stomach
2. Spleen/pancreas
3. Heart
4. Small intestine
5. Bladder
6. Kidneys
7. Circulation
8. Hormonal system
9. Gall bladder
10. Liver
11. Lungs
12. Colon

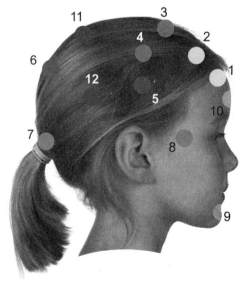

Carnial Lines and Points

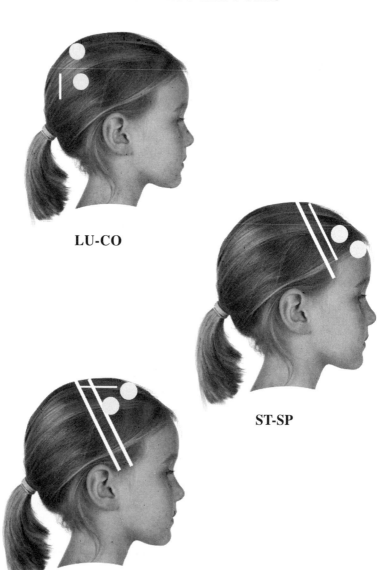

LU-CO

ST-SP

SI-H

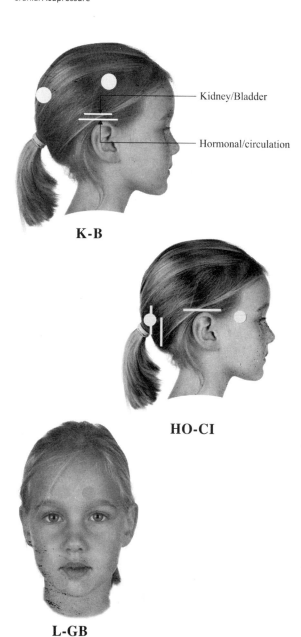

Kidney/Bladder

Hormonal/circulation

K-B

HO-CI

L-GB

Illustration: Cranial lines and points

The cranial points are connected directly to the brain center and the muscles of the body.

1. The Stomach point – The muscular group related to the Stomach meridian.

2. The Spleen/Pancreas point – The muscular group related to the Spleen/Pancreas meridian.

3. The Heart point – The muscular group related to the Heart meridian.

4. The Small intestine – The muscular group related to the Small intestine meridian.

5. The Bladder point – The muscular group related to the Bladder meridian.

6. The Kidney point – The muscular group related to the Kidney meridian.

7. The Blood circulation point – The muscular group related to the Circulation meridian.

8. The Hormonal point – The muscular group related to the Endocrine system meridian.

9. The Gall bladder point – The muscular group related to the Gall bladder meridian.

10. The Liver point – The muscular group related to the Liver meridian.

11. The Lung point – The muscular group related to the Lung meridian.

12. The Colon point – The muscular group related to the Colon meridian.

The cranial points and the lines on the cranium are stimulated according to the need of the patient. A point and a line can be stimulated in combination with the basic stimulation.

Similarly, all the points and lines can be stimulated individually or in combination with music and chromotherapy.

> *The scalp micro-system, which corresponds to the underlying somatosensory cerebral cortex, is the principal system in which the side of the microsystem reflex is contralateral to the side of body pathology.*

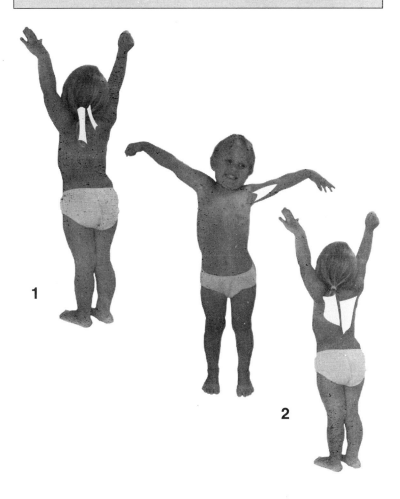

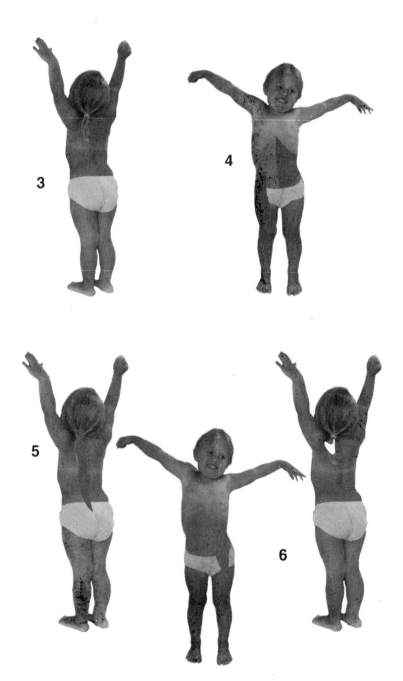

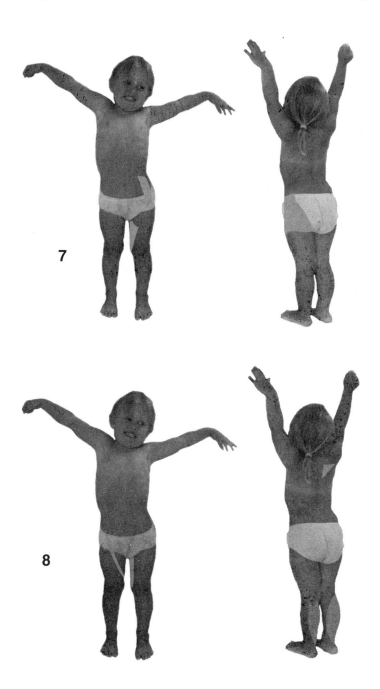

7

8

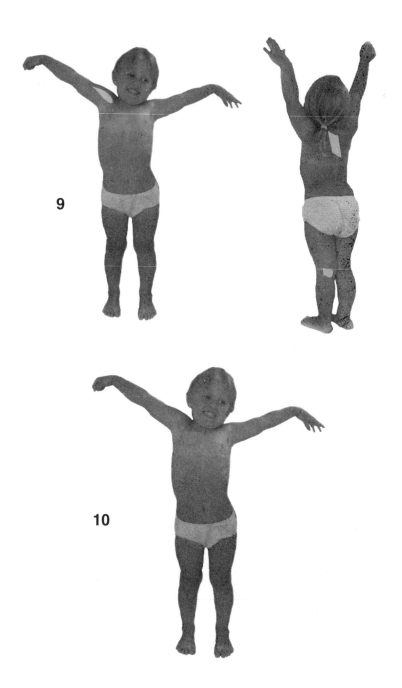

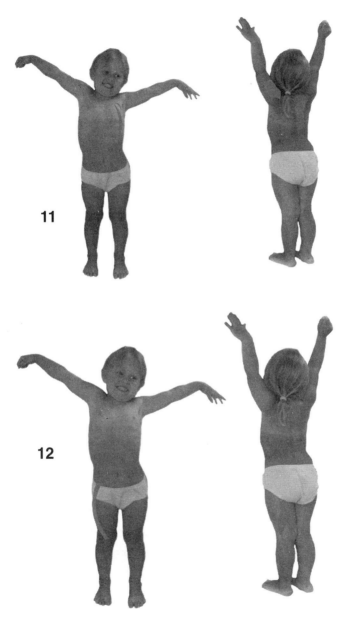

Illustration: *Cranial points in relation to muscles of the body*

Cranial Points: Colon / Lungs

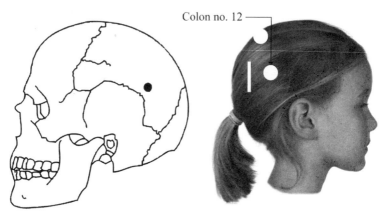

Colon no. 12

Relationship

Plexus	: Larynx
Zone of the body	: All the body
Attribute	: Bodily expression
Music	: Schubert

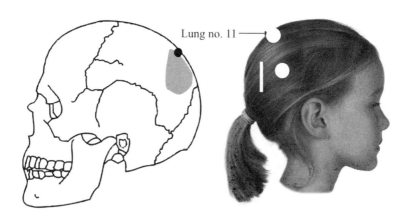

Lung no. 11

Illustration: *Cranial points – Colon / Lung*

Cranial Points: Stomach / Spleen

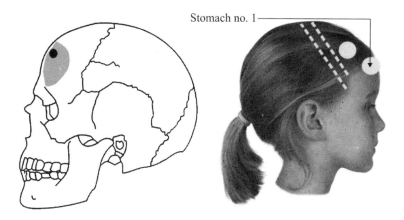

Stomach no. 1

Relationship

Plexus	:	Solar
Zone of the body	:	Thorax cavity, left side of the body
Attribute	:	Intelligence / Learning
Music	:	Verdi

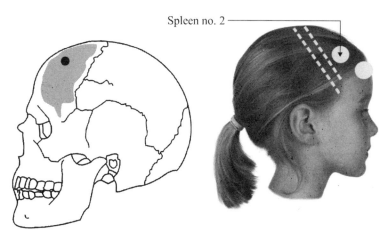

Spleen no. 2

Illustration: *Cranial points – Stomach / Spleen*

Cranial Points: Heart / Small Intestine

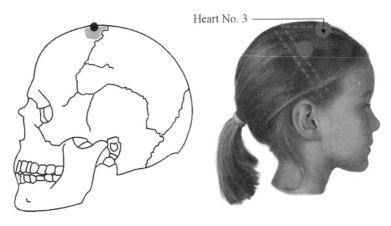

Relationship

Plexus	: Cardiac
Zone of the body	: Chest and head
Color	: Violet
Attribute	: Inspiration
Music	: Verdi

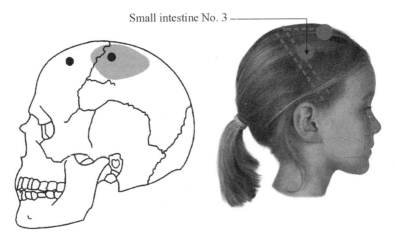

Illustration: *Cranial points – Heart/Small intestine*

Cranial Points: Kidney / Bladder

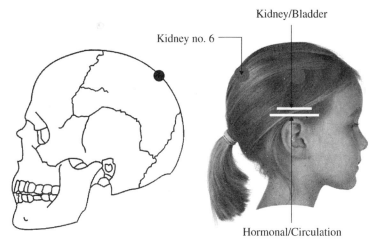

Kidney/Bladder

Kidney no. 6

Hormonal/Circulation

Relationship

Plexus	: Sacral
Zone of the body	: Abdomen
Attribute	: Vital strength
Music	: Mozart

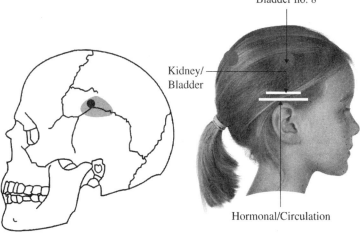

Bladder no. 8

Kidney/Bladder

Hormonal/Circulation

Illustration: *Cranial points – Kidney/Bladder*

Cranial Points: Hormonal / Blood Circulation

Harmonal no. 8 ——————

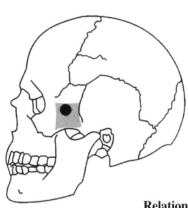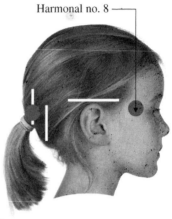

Relationship

Plexus   : Larynx
Zone of the body : All the body
Color   : Orange
Attribute   : Creative expression
Music   : Mozart

Circulation no. 9

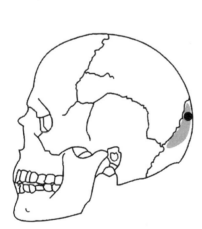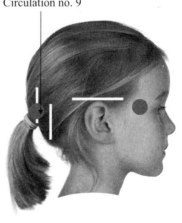

Illustration: Cranial points – Hormonal and Circulation

Cranial Points: Liver / Gall bladder

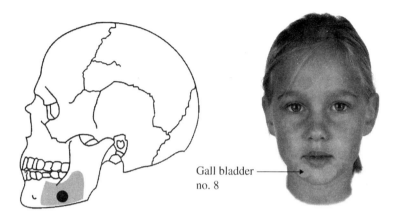

Gall bladder
no. 8

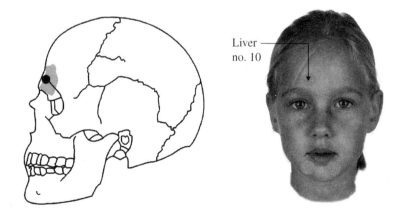

Liver
no. 10

Illustration: *Cranial points – Liver and Gall bladder*

Medical History

MEDICAL CASE RECORD

Name:	Medical history Nº

Date of birth: /   /
Address:
Code(   ) City   Country:
Home: Work: Mobile:
Symptoms:
Meridian:

Zone:
Grade:
Medication:
NP points:
Plexus:
Hormonal glands:
Vertebra:

Micro Model of the Brain Computer

MODEL OF COMPUTER STIMULATION

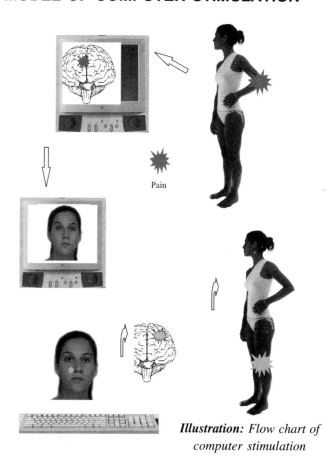

Illustration: *Flow chart of computer stimulation*

FUNCTIONAL AREAS OF THE CORTEX I

Location of the upper
body in the cortex

Location of the feet
and legs in the cortex

The arms and wrists are placed
in the lateral side of the brain.

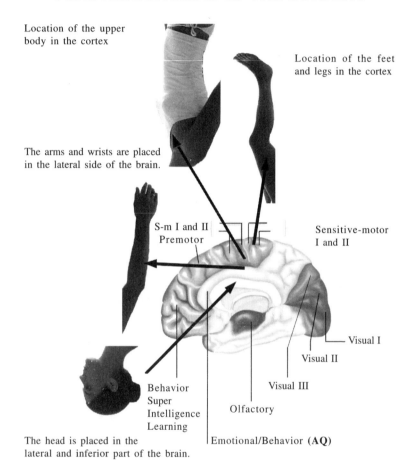

S-m I and II
Premotor

Sensitive-motor
I and II

Visual I

Visual II

Behavior
Super
Intelligence
Learning

Visual III

Olfactory

The head is placed in the
lateral and inferior part of the brain.

Emotional/Behavior (AQ)

Illustration: *Functional area of the cortex*

Representation of the Body on the Brain

A representation of the body exists in the neurons of the cerebral cortex, the subcortical thalamus and the reticular formation of the brain stem. This brain map has the same pattern as the map on the face representing the body.

Leg

Representation of the leg and foot on the superior and medial side of the cerebral cortex.

Arm

Representation of the arm and hand on the peripheral and lateral side of the cerebral cortex.

Head

Representation of the head on the most inferior and lateral side of the cerebral cortex.

The Cibernetic System

The 564 points that are presented here are nerve endings that branch out in the face. These points are scattered all over the body, but the ones that have been researched mainly on the face, were originally called *Cibernetic points* (points that cause a biofeedback effect). These points have a direct connection to centres of the brain that are incharge of organs, body functions and stimulate production of different chemicals like endorphins and pain blockers. Such points are used mainly to relieve symptoms, but some of them can also be used to support the balancing process that begins when we start working with the cause of the imbalance, that is, step number two. These points are very powerful and should not be used for long period of time, since they belong to the nervous system and an over stimulation might end in a lack of response. To use the points selected from the list given in this book, a very important and critical step should be taken into account called the stimulation of the 0 point. 0 point stimulation is in reality the stimulation of the limbic system, specifically an organelle called the amygdala. It is responsible for storing negative emotions that are necessary for survival, but the brain also uses it to store negative emotions that have been processed in a conscious manner. However, this might cause a lot of extra activity in the network of nerves, that might not allow the points to be stimulated efficiently or to reach the organ or brain centre that it was designed for. That is why the area of the 0 point is rubbed on both sides of the ear about 15 times (very close to the ears), in an up and down manner. This is done to stimulate the amygdala so that some of those negative emotions can be released, so there is no 'excessive traffic' in the brain and then proceed to stimulate the neurological points. This is also done when stimulation of these points are finished, since the effect of the 0 point stimulation and rubbing later, resets it to its normal state.

The amygdala is closely related to the sympathetic and parasympathetic system and too much activity in it causes an over stimulation in the sympathetic system, leading the body to be in a permanent stress state which is not beneficial for our health and so this is a crucial step every time some of the 564 points are used.

Central Nervous System – Regions of the Brain

Cortical brain regions: This highest level of the brain determines intellectual thinking, learning and memory, initiates voluntary movements and is consciously aware of sensations and feelings.

Pre-frontal cortex: This is the most evolved region of the human cortex and initiates conscious decisions.

Frontal cortex: This anterior cortical region contains the pre-central gyrus motor cortex which initiates specific, voluntary movements by activating upper motor neurons in the pyramidal system that sends direct neural impulses to lower motor neurons in the spinal cord.

Parietal cortex: This posterior region contains the post-central gyrus, the somatosensory cortex, which consciously perceives the sense of touch and spatial relationships.

Temporal cortex: This posterior and lateral cortical region contains the hearing centers of the brain. The left temporal lobe processes the verbal meaning of language and the rational logic of maths, whereas the right temporal lobe processes the intonation and rhythm of sounds.

Occipital cortex: This most posterior cortical region processes conscious and visual perceptions. The left occipital lobe can consciously read words, whereas the right occipital lobe is superior at recognizing faces and emotional expressions.

Corpus callosum: This broad band of myelinated axon fibers connect the left cerebral hemisphere cortical lobes with their respective lobe on the right cerebral hemisphere.

Cerebellum: This posterior region beneath the occipital lobe and above the pons is part of the extrapyramidal system and controls voluntary movements and postural adjustments.

Subcortical brain regions: These regions of the brain serve as an intermediary between the cerebral cortex above and the spinal cord below, operating outside of conscious awareness.

Thalamus: This spherical nucleus relays sensory messages from lower brainstem regions up to a specific locus on the cerebral cortex. The thalamus also contains neurons, which participate in the supra-spinal arousal of pain and in general arousal or sedation.

Ungulate cortex: This paleocortex limbic region lies beneath the neocortex.

Hippocampus: This semicircular limbic structure lies beneath the neocortex, but outside the thalamus. It affects attention span, long term memory storage and emotional experiences.

Posterior hypothalamus: This nucleus connects to the limbic system and the pituitary gland. It activates the sympathetic nervous system, producing general arousal and aggression.

Limbic system: This collection of subcortical nuclei affects emotions and memory.

Ungulate cortex: This paleocortex limbic region lies continuously beneath the neocortex.

Hippocampus: This semicircular limbic structure lies beneath the neocortex, but outside the thalamus. It affects attention span, long term memory storage and emotional experiences.

Amygdala nucleus: This spherical, limbic nucleus lies under the lateral, temporal lobe and modulates increases or decreases in aggressiveness, irritability and mania.

Septal nucleus: This medial limbic structure is involved in pleasure sensations and rewards.

Striatum: These basal ganglia nuclei lie along the limbic system, outside the thalamus. The specific striatal nuclei include the caudate, putamen, and globus pallidus, all of which are part of the extrapyramidal system control of semi-voluntary movements.

Brainstem: This term refers to the medulla oblongata, pons and midbrain altogether. It affects basic, unconscious control of body metabolism.

Pons: This brainstem region lies below the cerebellum and affects Rapid Eye Movement in sleep and dreams.

Midbrain tectum: This superior part of the midbrain contains colliculi for sensory reflexes.

Midbrain tegmentum: This inferior part of the midbrain affects basic metabolism and pain.

Reticular formation: This region within the midbrain tegmentum activates general arousal.

Red nucleus and substantia nigra: This region within the midbrain tegmentum affects the extrapyramidal system, the striatum and regulates semi-voluntary movements.

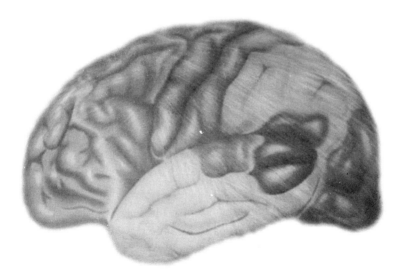

Illustration: Cortex of Brain

BRAIN CORTEX FUNCTIONAL AREAS II

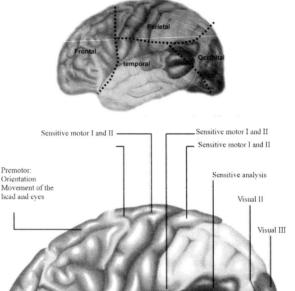

Sensitive motor I and II

Sensitive motor I and II
Sensitive motor I and II

Premotor:
Orientation
Movement of the
head and eyes

Sensitive analysis

Visual II

Visual III

Prefrontal:
Behavior
control
Superior
intelligence

Auditive I

Auditive II

Language
Reading
Speech

Visual I

Motor Control of
Speech

Illustration: *Brain cortex functional area II*

Frontal area : Planning and movement
(AQ)Parietal area: Somatic sensation
Temporal area: Hearing, memory, emotion and learning.
(AQ)Parietal area: Integration, body image
Occipital area: Primary visual receptor
Parietal-Temporal-Occipital area: Language

BRAIN CORTEX FUNCTIONAL AREAS

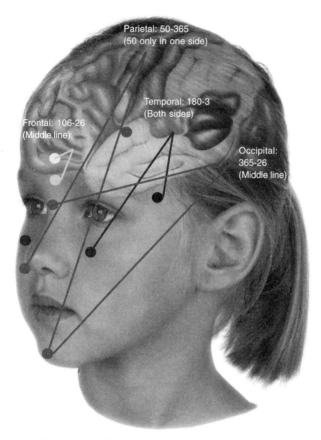

llustration: *Brain cortex functional area (AQ)*

Neurological points (page 182-184)
Parietal: Neurological points 50-365
Temporal: Neurological points 180-3
Occipital : Neurological points 365-8
Frontal: Neurological points 197-26

564 NEUROLOGICAL POINTS

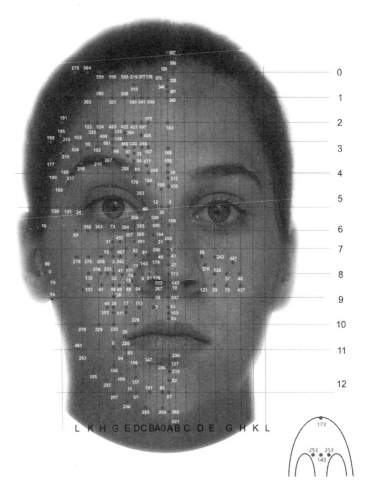

Illustration: 564 neurological points

1. Rub the area of the 0 point on both sides of the ear at the same time, about 15 times (the 0 points are very close to the ears), in an up and down manner.

2. Then press on the neurological point selected from the following lists, the lowest number and the highest number

for each of the problems that are required to be treated, **by applying pressure for 1 minute one by one.**

3. Finish the procedure by rubbing the area of the 0 point on both sides of the ear at the same time, about 15 times, in an up and down manner, as in step 1.

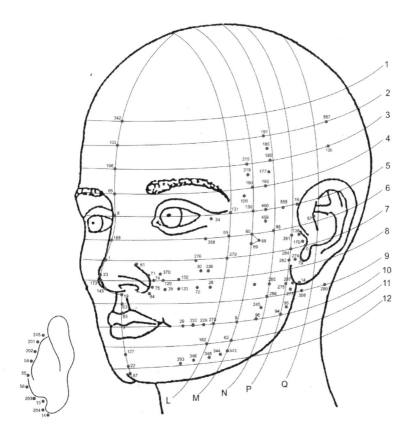

Illustration: 564 neurological points

Neurological Points Corresponding to the Different Areas of the Body

Head

Parietal region: 103-106-126-50-51-87-365.

Temporo-facial: 41-180-100-58-61-3-54-55.

Occipital: 106-564-26-65-188-87-365-127-8-290-100-139.

Frontal: 106-103-197-26-60-39-61-51.

Ears: 65-179-290-45-235-197-421-41.

Eyes: 103-197-16-34-188-50-3-20-6-105.

Nose: 126-184-65-26-61-39-50-3-197-555.

Lips / Mouth: 8-37-39-3-61.

Neck: 8-12-20-290-106-107.

Tongue: 8-312-79-57-60.

Teeth: 8-196-43-188-34-57-63-22-127.

Maxillary: 8-196-12-312-188.

Face: 60-57-37-58.

Upper Body

Shoulder: 477-106-107-310-34-97-98.

Shoulder's articulation: 88-564-278-559.

Arm: 97-98-99-267-360-60-0-51.

Elbow: 28-98-19-191.

Forearm: 324-129-217-60-0-51.

Wrist: 100-130-235-41-0.

Thumb: 61-180-3.

Index finger: 39-185.

Middle finger: 38-195-60.

Ring finger: 79-222-177.

Small finger: 191-6.

Lower Body

Pubic bone: 5-210-219-277.

Hip joint: 64-74-175.

Thighs: 9-17-113-37-38-50-3.

Knee: 29-222.

Knee-cap: 9-96-39-97-422-156-129.

Leg: 6-96-50-156-360.

Ankle: 347-107-310.

Foot: 34-51-127-461-107-310.

1. Toe: 34-127-51-461-107-310. (big toe)

2. Toe: 255-344.

3. Toe: 256-345.

4. Toe: 257-346.

5. Toe: 292-293.

Thorax

Rib cage: 189-73-467-491-13-269-3-60.

Breasts: 12-73-39-59-60.

Abdomen

Supraumbilical: 123-63-61-58-39-37-50.

Periumbilical: 63-53-59-222-127.

Infraumbilical: 127-87-235-22.

Back

Spine: 126-342-103-1-143-19-63.

Interscapular: 310-360-491-565.

Lumbosacral: 390-1-43-45-41-341-342-300-210-560

Organs

Skin and mucus membrane: 26-61-3-19-79.

Brain: 124-103-126-34-125-26-65.

Heart: 59-60-67-8-34-106-107-19-191.

Lung: 26-3-28-132-61-491-467-125.

Liver: 50-103-197-423-58-189-184.

Gall bladder: 41-184-139-54-55.

Spleen: 37-40-124.

Pancreas: 63-7-113.

Stomach: 39-120-121-37-50-61-5-45-21-63-19-127-210-54-55.

Small intestine: 127-22-34-348-8.

Colon: 342-561-98-19-17-143-38-9-104-105.

Kidney: 0-1-43-45-29-222-9-210-342-300-301-302.

Bladder: 85-87-22-235-26-126-29-3-89-60.

Uterus: 63-19-235-22-87.

Ovary: 7-113-287-65-73-156-347.

Penis and vagina: 19-63-1-50-0.

Testicle: 7-113-287-65-73-156.

Rectum: 19-143-126-365.

Plan of Worksheet for a Child with Learning Disabilities

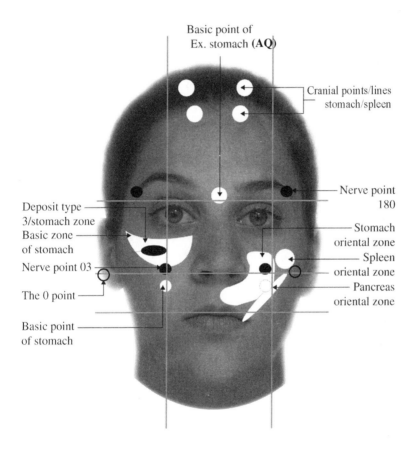

Illustration: *Worksheet for a child with learning disabilities*

Major deposit in the base of the stomach zone. Brain area corresponding to learning on the temporal cortex/points 3-180.

Worksheet Plan for The Treatment of An Ovary/ Deposit in The Hormonal Area Basic Zone

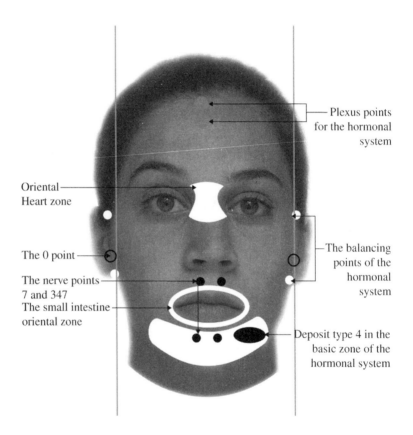

Plexus points for the hormonal system

Oriental Heart zone

The 0 point

The nerve points 7 and 347
The small intestine oriental zone

The balancing points of the hormonal system

Deposit type 4 in the basic zone of the hormonal system

Illustration: *Worksheet plan for the treatment of an ovary/deposit in hormonal area*

CHAPTER 15

Method of Reading the Face Visually

It is possible to analyse the face by observing stigmas or changes in the face of the patient.

Depending on intensity of the problem, the face can reveal the patient's status of health. The coloring and texture of the skin whether it be pale or the opposite, a flushed or discolored complexion with an increase in the vascularization, moles, vitiligo, small nodules and open pores.

1. Lung zone: White, pale, transparent with broken capillaries.
2. Colon zone: Deep wrinkle in the zone with the tissue being very thin.
3. Hormonal zone: Red, inflamed acne.
4. Stomach zone: Yellow and inflamed.
5. Spleen zone: Fragile and delicate skin which is yellow in color.
6. Kidney zone: Dark and thin tissue.
7. Liver and Gall bladder: Green, with deep wrinkles on the forehead between the eyes.
8. Heart zone: Point of the nose red and inflamed. Zone just above the eyebrow is swollen.
9. Bladder zone: Swollen and white.
10. Small intestine zone: Red with dry skin.

Evaluating the state of health of the patient is done by a combination of visual observations and analysis carried through a touch of fingers.

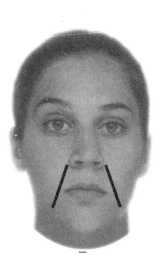

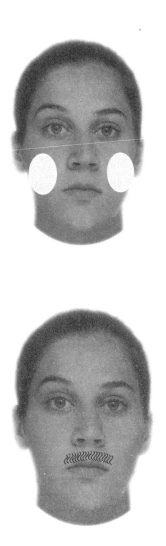

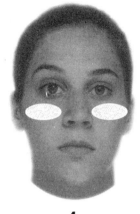

4

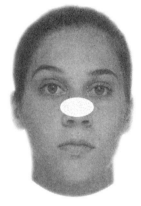

5

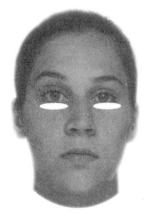

6

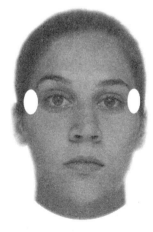

7

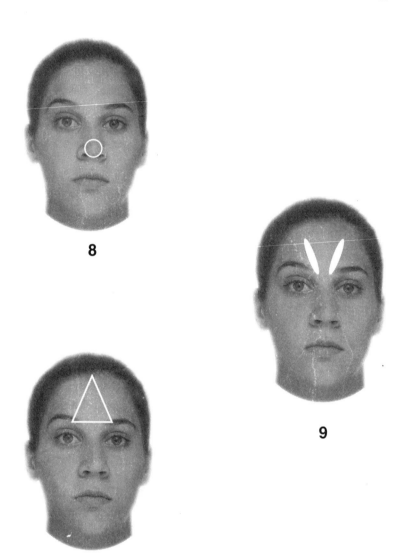

Illustration: The areas used to visually observe the functioning of the
vital organs

Chapter 16

Neurovascular Points for Wrinkles

POINTS FOR WRINKLES

By observing the wrinkles and creases in the face it is possible to determine the state of degeneration of the organ corresponding to the respective zone. The illustration shows the relevant points to be stimulated in accordance with the location of the wrinkles on the face.

Es/n. 73
Co/n. 113
Gob/n.63
Co/n.63
Cen/n.286

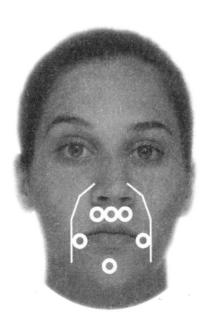

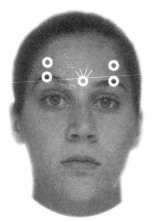

V/n.428
V/n.267
Hi/n.26

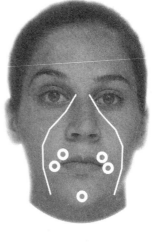

Co/n. 113
Co/n.222
Cen/n.286

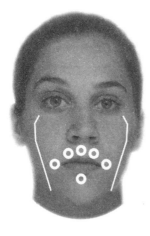

Gob/n.63
Co/n.113
Cen/n.286
Co/n.113

The points for wrinkles can be treated by pressing your fingertips and giving a circular massage 8-10 times on each point or the points can be treated with bio-lazer for 1 minute.

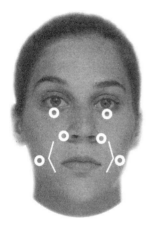

Co/n.229
Es/n.73

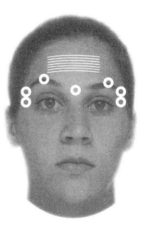

3E/n.218
3E/n.217
V/n.267
Hi/n.108

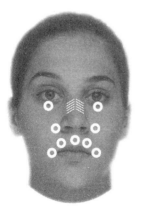

Es/n.73
Co/n.27
Gob/n.63
Co/n.113
Co/n.223

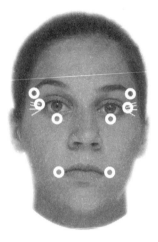

3E/n.217
3E/n.231
Es/n.17
Co/n.222

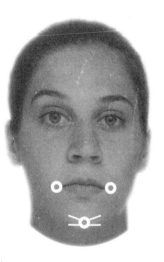

Co/n.222
Cen/n.286
Gob/n.521

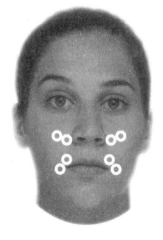

Co/n.32
Co/n.75
Co/n.228
Co/n.222

Illustration: Points for wrinkles

This book is a presentation of the Facial Reflexology base system and four additional methods.

The full Facial Reflexology concept contains 10 other additional facial reflex methods to add to the base treatment and are used to treat patients for individual and personal problems.

Yamamoto Cranial therapy

Dr Wong chines acupressure therapy

Colonlink method

NP individual therapy

Cyber therapy self-treatment

Labour/birth stimulation

Emotional stimulation

Method for children's therapy

Esthetical use of Facial Reflexology

Japanese face lifting method

CHAPTER 17

CASES AROUND THE WORLD
(Case Histories written by students)

Patient's Age : School going girl

Diseases: Migraine and Nausea

Therapist : Akiko, Osaka, Japan.

Result: I treated Moe, two times last week.

She looked fine, slept well, her eyes looks stronger and more shining!

When school started, Moe was happy to go back to school.

She no longer complained of migraine and nausea anymore.

Fourth report about Moe from Japan:

I treated Moe twice, and I asked, Moe's mother to continue additional stimulations every day.

This morning Moe's mother called me and told me that Moe's skin condition has improved a lot after stimulating the new points/ combination.

Before, Moe had very dry and itchy skin during winter, and it was getting drier and drier since last month. However, this week it suddenly got better.

Also, she is no longer suffering from constipation. She had been suffering from constipation since she was baby.

Now I'm expecting a good effect on her eyes too.

Patient's Age : 78 year Male

Diseases: Stroke Mood swings Speech loss Memory loss

Therapist : Akiko, London, UK

Result: Today, I started using Tibetan reflex therapy front and scalp technique for my client who had a stroke 10 years ago in 1999.

Symptom: Mood swings, speech loss, memory loss.

Medication: Anti-depressive medication (2 types) from August 2009, four other medication for high cholesterol.

In October 2009, I started treating him weekly for 7 sessions. Restarted treatment every fortnight since March 2010.

His speech has improved and now he is able to speak longer sentences and much more clearer. He has no more temper, is calm. Also, last week the doctor told him that he doesn't need to take any anti-depressive medication any more! What great news!!

He is very very happy receiving Facial reflex therapy. I'll continue treating him and I'll let you know the progress.

Patient's Age : 56 year Male

Diseases: Muscular sclerosis Fibromyalgia and Squamous cell carcinoma Throat cancer (remission since 2004)

Therapist : Allisson Parks Barne, NC, USA

Result: Medical history of muscular sclerosis, fibromyalgia, squamous cell carcinomas, throat cancer (remission since 2004).

Medications: Hydrocodone (for pain), Avenex (for muscular sclerosis), Flexeril (a muscle relaxant) and multivitamins.

SESSION ONE:

Complaint today: Low back pain.

Patient was much more relaxed after the session and no longer low back pain.

SESSION TWO:

Complaint today: Low back pain but less than before; pain in right wrist and feeling of less energy.

Patient was much more relaxed after the session; the low back pain had eased but was still sore; there was less pain in the right wrist and he was able to rotate his hand.

SESSION THREE:

Complaint today: Indigestion, pain in the neck.

Patient stated that he had been feeling a lot better with little to no pain. He felt more energetic too. Patient was much more relaxed after the session; felt less tension in the neck and complained of no indigestion at the time.

SESSION FOUR:

Complaint today: Mild lower back pain, pain in the neck, mild headache.

Patient stated he felt that his balance was better since the last treatment.

He has not had any low back pain or headache since last treatment.

SESSION FIVE:

Complaint today: Patient has no pain today, just a mild tension in the neck. Patient is feeling a lot better and has more energy. There is an overall feeling of well being.

Patient's Age : 30 year Female

Diseases: Milk production (increasing)

Therapist : Ania, Poland

Result: Here is a wonderful experience of increasing milk production with facial reflexology. It is an interesting case because the Japanese woman, said that in Japan it is very popular, but she didn't try it. It was funny that she had she had the popular treatment of Japan in Poland.

Patient's Age : 36 year Male

Diseases: Irritable bowel syndrome (IBS)

Therapist : Anu Laatikainen, Abu Dhabi, UAE

Result: Symptoms: Suffering from IBS, no medication; mainly stress related (work), does lots of running but gets pain in his knee after training.

AFTER EIGHTH TREATMENT:

Treatment as previously; found his skin looking healthier. Client relaxed throughout the session. He informs that his stomach/ digestive system has been much better; IBS symptoms have calmed down a lot. Also, his knee pain has reduced. He was very satisfied with his treatment as he was always feeling very relaxed and sleepy during and after the session. Client almost always complained of headache after every session which gave me some reassurance that he was responding to the sessions.

Patient's Age : 30 year Female

Diseases: Pelvic discomfort/ heaviness

Therapist : Anu Laatikainen, Abu Dhabi, UAE

Result: Symptoms: Pregnant with her second child; due date 1.4.2010. No medical problems noted before or during her pregnancy. She is suffering from pelvic discomfort/heaviness at the moment. Has never had an alternative therapy during her pregnancy. Medication: Antenatal vitamins.

Client enjoyed her treatment and was feeling more relaxed afterwards.

EIGHTH TREATMENT/39 WEEKS

Client has been feeling very restless today and has been getting stronger tightenings. I was able to palpate her tightenings clearly.

They were coming irregularly and lasting only 15 seconds. The tightenings were not painful at all.

After 48 hours of the last treatment, the client started having regular/painful contractions; she was able to stay at home during the first part of the labor and went to hospital when having contractions less than 5 minutes apart. Two hours later she had normal/ uncomplicated spontaneous vaginal delivery; just using entonox.

Baby girl 3.4 kg! I went to see the mother and baby the same evening in the hospital. The mother was feeling very happy and energetic. She was amazed how less tired she was after this delivery and how smoothly and quickly everything happened, in comparison to her first delivery. She is bonding very well with her baby who was breastfeeding with no problems.

The client was very happy with the course of treatment she had during the last two months of her pregnancy. She feels that the sessions have helped her to be more balanced with the different changes of her pregnancy. Also she generally felt less discomfort during this delivery time than with her first pregnancy.

This case study also gave me lots of knowledge regarding how facial reflexology works for pregnant woman and to study more and use this skills for other pregnant women.

Patient's Age : 3 year old girl

Diseases: Asthma/ Eczema

Therapist : Bauke, Netherlands

Result: Frequently suffers from infections, colds.

The client was given a combination of face and neuro/foot reflex therapy as the girl could not lie still for so long.

After first treatment more eczema as a reaction of treatment.

I treated her for 3 months, giving one session a week. She never had an attack of asthma during this time.

She had difficulty in breathing only once in these 3 months and there were no infections also, She only had one attack of only cold.

Patient's Age : 1.5 year old girl

Diseases: Ear infections

Therapist : Bauke, Netherlands

Result: Already suffered from ear infections 8 times for which she has received antibiotics 8 times. Also often complains of running nose.

She did not like treatments on the face. So I treated her with neuro – foot reflexology including extra maps for the ears, nose, thymus and tonsils on the toes area. I gave a map of points for the ears so her mother could do some extra work at home. I did 7 sessions in total, once a week. I treated her father with facial reflexology for headaches caused by stress and eating a lot of chocolate. He still comes (3, 5 years) once a month to relax. His daughter is now almost 5 years old and she has never had an ear infection again.

Patient's Age : 27 year Female

Diseases: Facial paralysis for 1 week (Bells syndrome)

Therapist : Bauke, Netherlands

Result: Doctor told her to get foot reflexology! I did facial reflexology instead. After 8 sessions she looked almost normal again. After 12 sessions, her facial nerve as totally normal. When she are suffering from stress her face become a little stiff again, but then she just took an extra session and she is fine again.

Patient's Age : 29 year Female

Diseases: Facial paralysis for 16 days (Bells syndrome)

Therapist : Bauke, Netherlands

Result: I did facial reflexology. After 2 or 3 sessions, her face looked almost normal again. It was only when she smiled that her mouth became crooked. After the fifth session, she went back to working. A week later, she underevent a lot of stress. This made her mouth and eye a bit crooked again. I started giving her sessions, twice a week for 3 weeks after which she was okay. Her face was totally normal. I talked to her a few weeks ago, 4 months after the treatment and it's still good.

Patient's Age : 46 year Female

Diseases: Hyper-ventilation

Therapist : Bauke, Netherlands

Result: The patient suffered from (3 years) hyper-ventilation, no attacks but very subtle but constant hyper-ventilation. She always had a sensation of pressure on the chest; she sighed a lot all day and complained of fatigue. The doctor could not do anything. She practiced yoga for 6 years but it did not help her. She also tried acupuncture, physiotherapy and osteopathy; all these alternative therapies did not help her. I did facial reflexology.

During one session I noticed that she did not sigh so much anymore, her breathing was almost normal. After 9 sessions she was feeling fine. I gave her some homework – to work on some points on the face at home.

After 6 sessions at home, she felt much better; she could enjoy life more now, especially the small things in life. She felt happy again, she had not felt this way for years. She still comes to me once a month for a session since the last 4 years now.

Patient's Age : 35 year Female

Diseases: Insomnia Wish to get pregnant again

Therapist : Bauke, Netherlands

Result: A lady had a miscarriage followed by the birth of a little girl, which was again followed by a miscarriage. This was a couple of weeks before I started the treatment. After 1 session of facial reflexology she become pregnant and the pregnancy went well. She delivered a healthy boy. Her sleep pattern was also better. I gave her four sessions in all.

Patient's Age : 1 year old girl

Diseases: Insomnia

Therapist : Bauke, Netherlands

Result: The girl could neither sleep well at night nor during the day. She does not like to be alone or play alone; she always wanted to be with her mother. She was one of a twin, her twin sister died during the pregnancy. She did not like to be treated on the face so I did neuro foot reflexology.

In total I gave her 6 sessions, but after the first session she woke only once in the night, and she slept better after every treatment.

Patient's Age : 36 year Female

Diseases: Migraine

Therapist : Bauke, Netherlands

Result: Sometimes she had the migraine attack several times a month, one attack following the other, and at other times a couple of month's go by without any attack. When she has migraine she is sick a couple of days. She has to lie down in a dark room; it is accompanied by vomiting. I treated her with facial reflexology. In the beginning, the attack of migraines occured more frequently and more intensity, later they occured without vomiting. After 10 sessions, there were no more attacks of migraine. She comes for treatment now once every 2 or 3 months as maintenance. She had an attack of migraine only once when she had a lot of stress.

Patient's Age : 38 year Female

Diseases: Migraine for 6 years

Therapist : Bauke, Netherlands

Result: Really sick every 2 or 3 weeks. Facial reflexology was given sometimes along with neuro foot reflexology. After 7 sessions she had no migraine anymore. However, sometimes she companied of a headache. After 11 session, there were no more headaches.

Patient's Age : 51 year Female

Diseases: Migraine since childhood

Therapist : Bauke, Netherlands

Result: After one session she had migraine lasting for 3 days but for only 2 hours a day. Normally her migraine attack lasted 2 or 3 days constantly. After that she did not have migraine again. I gave her 9 sessions and she told me that she would come back if she had an attack of migraine again. I never heard from her again, it's been 2 years now.

Patient's Age : 68 year Male

Diseases: Phlegm in sinuses

Therapist : Bauke, Netherlands

Result: The patient did not have a cold or any pain; only his voice had changed and he could not smell. His doctor gave him medicine but the medicine did not help him, so the doctor wanted to operate on him. My patient does not want to undergo surgery because he knew someone who did have a surgery which ended in brain damage because of the operation. He asked the doctor to wait a couple of months and decided to try facial reflexology in the mean time. I treated him with facial reflexology and neuro foot reflexology. After 4 sessions the phlegm was reduced. After 7 sessions he started to smell again and he felt more energy. The doctor then delayed the surgery. After 16 sessions, his sinuses were clean and did not need an operation.

Diseases: Mental retardation

Therapist : Beijing, China

Result: Mentally retarded children were shown to improve significantly in height, weight, health states, social living abilities and intellectual development when receiving foot reflexology as opposed to those not receiving treatment.

Diseases: Brain damage/ Aneurysms

Therapist : Lone Sorensen, Denmark Written by Berit Skrumsager, Denmark (Mother of Justin)

Result: JUSTIN'S CASE – BRAIN DAMAGE

"When are you coming home daddy?" Those were Justin's very first words in his life, spoken when he was 6 years old. Justin had brain damage since infancy and thanks to his mother, Berit Skrumsager's patient training with Temprana reflex therapy, he is now able to talk.

When the journalist visited Justin and his family 4 years later, Justin stood in the doorway, ready to reach out, shake hands and say "Hi" to any visitor to his family home, a cozy little house situated in Bronshoj, a suburb of Copenhagen.

The 10 year old smiles widely as he says with perfect clarity, "Look at my trampoline in the backyard, I just love it!"

In the family's living room a child-sized wheelchair stands neglected in the corner, while the centre of the room is dominated by a lawn lounge chair that plays a very important role in Justin's life but we'll come back to that later.

The little boy's brain damage is not immediately apparent, and only becomes obvious as his parents – Berit and Mark Skrumsager relate his life story.

Justin, who is Berit and Mark's third son, had a perfectly normal birth but, "A week after he was born we were concerned that his behavior was a little abnormal. He wouldn't suckle; when he was encouraged to feed he would just turn his head away," recalls Berit.

During the night his condition deteriorated and the following day he was taken by an ambulance to Copenhagen's main hospital emergency room. Justin was immediately admitted to the hospital's neonatal department. By this time he was breathing irregularly and he was suffering from cramps.

Further examination revealed that Justin had suffered a number of aneurysms that resulted in an accumulation of blood in his brain, and as his father Mark says, "That's when Justin's brain was damaged."

Berit continues, "After a day and a half in the hospital, the doctors told us that the chances of Justin surviving past the age of 3 months were about 50 per cent. We decided then and there to discharge him, and take him home with us – we thought that if he was going to die, we would rather have him be at home."

All that Berit and Mark could do now was to wait and hope for the best. They each had their own ways of coping with the long and distressing wait.

A DIFFICULT TIME

Berit, who is a radiographer says, "I just had to concentrate on practical things. In my daily work I dealt with seriously ill people, so it wasn't unusual for me to think about dealing with death."

Mark joins in, "It was difficult for me. The entire period seemed surreal, I felt detached, and I kept thinking how unjust it was that our newborn son should have to suffer so much."

Both parents were overjoyed when they could see that Justin's condition gradually improved.

The baby was obviously afflicted by his condition, but he was nowhere near to being the 'vegetable' that the doctors had prepared Berit and Mark to expect.

Being the parents of a disabled child was something that they now had to mentally prepare themselves for. "In the following years, the biggest obstacle that we encountered was communicating with Justin. He used his body language whenever he wanted to tell us something, but it was far from being a big success, we didn't always notice – and because Justin doesn't have an aggressive nature, when he was sad or upset he would turn into himself – it was so frustrating for him."

Justin is normally so quiet and mild natured, that when he falls and hurts himself he goes into 'lock-down mode' that means that he stays where he's fallen and doesn't make a sound, even if the blood is gushing out of him. He falls over a lot because he walks on the tips of his toes. He has difficulty managing stairs or getting up again if he has been sitting on the floor.

Berit explains that in many ways, Justin is just like a little baby.

For the first time, in 2002, a friend of Berit's told her about a program called Temprana reflex therapy. "As a mother to a disabled child, I was open to all possibilities but I wouldn't go along with just anything," she says.

THE FIRST WORDS

Berit explains that Temprana reflex therapy is similar to standard foot reflexology, except that it is also performed on the face and hands, and more related to the nerve system.

Justin had a tailor made treatment program put together specifically for his condition and Berit was trained to personally treat her son. After bathing Justin in the evenings, she puts on a soothing music CD. Justin gets himself comfortable in the previously mentioned lawn lounge chair (which Berit has discovered is ideally suited to the purpose). "He just loves it and often falls asleep during the treatment which takes an hour," she says with a smile.

Berit noticed that Justin improved very quickly with the new Temprana treatment, "Suddenly he could perform a lot of ordinary little tasks such as pouring milk into a glass."

After a year and a half there was a major breakthrough.

Berit continues, "Mark phoned home from Dubai, where he was working at the time. Justin took the telephone and asked in a clear and perfectly understandable voice, "When are you coming home daddy?" Those were the very first words we had heard Justin say in his life; both Mark and I cried tears of joy."

In the period after that, Mark and Berit found themselves constantly and joyfully amazed by his progress.

"Justin's ability to talk completely changed our lives. The quality of our lives vastly improved, even now when we think back on it we can't help but beam with joy."

Berit still uses Temprana reflex therapy on Justin and intends to continue, she has a goal – she wants Justin to be toilet trained before he reaches puberty. This is possible with Temprana therapy, as it is normal to change to different programs when a goal is obtained.

Berit often meets skepticism when she talks about the treatment.

"People often ask me how I know that it is definitely Temprana reflex therapy that has helped my son. They speculate that Justin might just have developed that way anyway, but I have no doubt that Temprana reflex therapy is responsible. When using Temprana reflex therapy, we work with accepted and proven acupuncture points and nerve points, there is no hocus-pocus involved," says Berit.

One of the main reasons that Berit and Mark are so relieved with Justin's ability to speak is that they now know Justin will be more able to take care of himself when they are no longer there to care for him. Berit, who is now 48 years old used to be plagued with anxiety, "I used to worry constantly about how Justin would cope, should anything unexpected happen to Mark and myself, then I had a few sessions with a psychologist and that helped."

Berit and Mark are very good at communicating with each other and the Skrumsager family has been strengthened by the adversity they have had to deal with.

Both parents agree "We love Justin above all else, he's our little star, he's always so funny, positive and charming and a joy to be with."

Patient's Age : 6 year old boys and girls

Diseases: Children with special needs

Therapist : Charter School, UK

Result: December 2006 Review of Complementary Therapy; Facial Reflexology at Charter School / 6 year old children with special needs:

Our continued objectives are: To help support the mental, physical, emotional and spiritual well being of the students.

We aimed to help improve the following:

1.   Self-esteem and confidence.

2.   Capacity to learn by improving attention span and concentration

3.   Calm hyperactivity by helping reduce tension and anxiety.

We also aimed to support and address the emotional needs and aspects of the children s development through puberty.

SUMMARY

20 Children Treated:

The majority of students have continued to respond well to the treatment. Our perception from the feedback we have received is that their behavior has improved; they are also calmer and more attentive in lessons. Most importantly, we feel the therapeutic relationship built between us and the students has become an important part of their school life, they feel able to confide in us, discuss some of their problems and air their views of how they feel about school. All the children without exception have said they all sleep much better (we had noticed during the summer break that their sleep patterns were disrupted). As therapists we continue to thoroughly enjoy the challenge and would like to treat more students with the available time slots as we feel there are more students in the school who could benefit from the treatment.

Patient's Age : 6 year old boys and girls

Diseases: ADHD and Autism (Results of a project)

Therapist : Charter School, UK

Result: July 2006 Review of Complementary Therapy at Charter School:

Our objectives are:

To help support the mental, physical, emotional and spiritual well being of students aged 6 years with ADHD and autism.

We aimed to help improve the following:

1.   Self-esteem and confidence.

2.   Capacity to learn by improving attention span and concentration.

3.   Calm hyperactivity by helping to reduce tension and anxiety.

We also aimed to support and address the emotional needs and aspects of the children s development through puberty.

CONCLUSION

We feel the pilot scheme has proven to be a very valuable exercise, which has benefited all the students in some way. Obviously some have responded quicker than others but as we regard each as an individual so we would expect our degree of success to vary accordingly. We believe that we have achieved some fantastic results in a very short time (but there is a lot more to be done!) Akeem s statement sums up for us better than we could have hoped how powerful and effective this treatment can be in helping children with special needs to cope with the challenges set before them. We feel this treatment can really help address the children s emotional needs which are not possible in any other way.

As therapists we have thoroughly enjoyed the challenge. We absolutely love working with the children and building the therapeutic relationship. It has been a real privilege and very rewarding to watch how they have responded to the treatments.

We very much hope that the Charter will allow us to continue this valuable work next term. As I mentioned, Professor George Ellison at St George's University London has agreed, subject to sourcing the funding to establish a full research study fully supported by the University. This will entail submitting an 80 page submission to the Department of Health Ethics Committee prior to the research project starting. I hope you will agree this would be a unique and groundbreaking opportunity for the school and it enables us to continue to give complementary therapy to children who would not normally be able to access such treatments.

Patient's Age : 82 year Female

Diseases: Rheumatoid arthritis

Therapist : Cheryl, Wales, UK

Result: The patient I'm treating with facial reflexology was crippled with rheumatoid arthritis. The patient s posture resembled a crab or a spider, as she was doubled over, that is, her back wasn't straight, her legs were wide apart, and her knees were bent outwards which forced her to walk with her feet out to the sides. On taking off the patient s shoes, I found that her toes were crossed.

From the first session, 2 nurses had to assist her to get the patient onto my couch to make the patient comfortable for me, so I didn't see her feet. I gave the patient a full facial reflexology treatment. The patient thoroughly enjoyed her treatment.

The following week, on visiting the patient for her second session, I found that her posture resembled a jockey; she looked as if she had just dismounted from a horse. She was more upright and her legs were better aligned, although the knees were still bent out to the side. One nurse came to assist in helping the patient onto my couch, so again I didn't see her feet. Everyone in the house was talking about the improvements to the patient s mobility.

After 3 weeks, there was even more improvement. I was able to help the patient up from her chair, and managed on my own, to get her onto my couch. Her feet were quite puffy and purple in color.

After 4 weeks, on visiting the lady, once again, I found a strong improvement in her posture. She no longer resembles a jockey, although her knees are slightly out of alingment. She now walks with her feet in a straight line, not pointing out to the side, and her mobility is amazing. On helping the patient onto my couch and taking off her shoes, I noticed that only one toe is crossed that being the toe next to the big toe, which is crossed on the middle joint, and all the purple discoloration had vanished. I called the Matron to come and see the patient's feet, and she was amazed.

After 5 weeks of session, this visit was the most exiting, as all her toes were straight. I was so amazed by how quickly this correction happened. I called the Matron home to see the patient s toes again.

The Matron came and said that she had never seen anything like this.

Patient's Age : 49 year old

Diseases: Psycotic schizophrenia Temporary

Therapist : Claris, Canada

Result: My patient, who was diagnosed with temporary psychotic schizophrenia is off her medication and is recovering very well. I will continue with facial reflexology sessions.

Patient's Age : 69 year Male

Diseases: Stroke

Therapist : Claris, Canada

Result: The stroke client I am still working with is doing well.

I added muscle stimulation to the treatment plan and with one session only his facial muscles, particularly on the left (paralysed side) 'relaxed.' His face looks better and has a healthy complexion. Also, as a result of his rehabilitation, oxygen treatment and facial reflex therapy, he no longer uses a wheel chair but uses a regular cane for walking. What tremendous progress... thanks to your continued support. I am so excited and happy.

Patient's Age : 56 year Female

Diseases: Anxiety/ Depression

Therapist : Connie NC, USA

Result: Complaint:

The woman suffered from severe anxiety and depression. She was on prescription medication to help her with these problems. The woman says that she often feels aches all over.

Conclusion: After the first session itself, the woman felt better. After 6 sessions, she reported that she no longer took anti-anxiety medication. The woman says that she is feeling better, is happier and no longer feels aches throughout the body. She will continue her sessions every 2 to 4 weeks with facial reflexology.

Patient's Age : 89 year Male

Diseases: Legs heavy

Therapist : Connie NC, USA

Result: Former professional tennis player.

Complaint: The legs felt heavy, he is unable to play tennis at the level he is used to. Sometimes it seemed as if his legs are not working properly. The man has had this problem since the past few months.

Conclusion: After 3 sessions, the client reported that he felt much better and is now able to play better tennis. His balance and movements are also much better.

Patient's Age : 53 year Female

Diseases: Arthritis (psoriatic)

Therapist : Connie, NC, USA

Result: A woman, 53 years old reports that she is having swelling in her joints. The swelling started in the knee and great toe of the left leg and spread to the left wrist, the right thumb and the right elbow.

SESSION 5: October 16, 2009 Client states that she was feeling 'pretty good' today. Her knee is better and she can walk better. The swelling in her feet is almost gone and she can wear regular shoes now but she still has some pain in the foot. Client still complains of pain in her wrist, down through her thumb. Client is in a good mood and happy with her progress.

The client is pleased with her progress and will continue to come for facial reflexology sessions once a week.

Patient's Age : 49 year Female

Diseases: Shoulder/Neck pain Hot flashes Insomnia Anxiety

Therapist : Connie, NC, USA

Result: Profession: Personal trainer and manager at a fitness center.

Complaint: Pain in the shoulder and neck, hot flashes, insomnia, anxiety.

Conclusion: After one session neck and shoulder pain disappeared. After two sessions hot flashes stopped and the client is sleeping better. The client will continue monthly for maintenance and to avoid any new symptoms that may occur.

Patient's Age : 64 year Female

Diseases: Sinuitis

Therapist : Connie, NC, USA

Result: Profession: Professional singer.

Complaint: The woman complained that her sinuses always feel 'full', her neck and her face feels swollen and puffy. On the second visit she complained also of pain in the shoulder, which prevented her from playing tennis.

Conclusion: After one session the woman reported that her sinuses were much better and that she could feel a big difference in the tone and resonance when she sang. The woman reported that her discomfort had disappeared days after the treatment. She would continue face reflexology session regularly (monthly).

Patient's Age : 52 year Male

Diseases: Tinnitus for the last 32 years

Therapist : Connie, NC, USA

Result: Client has suffered from severe tinnitus for the last 32 years.

The client has had multiple head traumas over the years for about 20 years ago, he suffered a gun shot wound right next to his head and ear. His tinnitus was so disturbing that he sometimes just sat in a corner, isolated from the outside world (shut himself away). The client suffered from chronic neck pain since the last 10 years.

Conclusion: After 20 sessions, the client reports that the tinnitus has reduced; it is now bearable, sometimes not even noticeable. The man says that the pain in his neck has disappeared and he now has full motion in his neck.

Patient's Age : 79 year Female

Diseases: Stroke

Therapist : Cyndi Hill , North Carolina, USA

Result: Update from a stroke patient.

The lady's family moved her to North Carolina (NC) after a stroke in the parietal lobe. There was weakness of muscles and the voice had no strength or volume. Initially, she had problem tracking with eyes, but that had cleared by the time she got to me. She also suffered from neuropathy prior to the stroke.

SESSION 1:

Feet were very tender. Could barely stand the lightest touch.

SESSION 2:

Voice much stronger. Quick witted. Loved facial reflexology, fascinated by hand reflexology though was still dreading foot reflexology. Adjusted pressure, praxis vertebralis and encouraged her to communicate with me on sensitivity levels.

Today her family brought her to church (this is a big deal!). She was bright eyed and coherent. She enjoyed conversing with everyone and is looking forward to her next session.

Patient's Age : 4 year old boy

Diseases: Down syndrome

Therapist : Cyndi Hill, North Carolina, USA

Result: Mother reports his vocabulary is increasing daily. Is better able to understand and follow directions. Was able to understand and comply with instructions to sit still for a haircut. I know it seems small, but mother was elated as this had not occurred before.

This will prove to be the most powerful tool parents have to help their children achieve their maximum potential. Pass the word along.

About my little Down's boy – his teeth were grinding, which is now almost completely stopped; vocabulary continues to increase; his skills in cooperation and understanding directions continue to develop.

Patient's Age : 58 year Female

Diseases: Pain in legs and feet Hot flashes Night sweats Insomnia

Therapist : David Henry, NC, USA

Result: Symptoms: Pain in lower leg and feet – calcification at proximal calcaneus – sensitivity in the Gastroc-nemius muscle. There is a thick congestion that accumulates around the proximal calcaneus – lateral and medial to the achilles tendon. The congestion is firm but can be manipulated and disperses after repeated foot reflexology. She says her 'calf muscles' are usually tender to touch. Client says that she feels that her overweight condition contributes to her sensitive feet and lower leg problems. Also, what she characterizes as pre-menopausal symptoms including hot flashes, night sweats and insomnia.

Notes: Client has seen a doctor of Oriental medicine on four occasions for acupuncture.

The doctor says she has 'limited chi in the spleen meridian' and that her gall bladder 'does not produce.' The congestion in her feet diminished during these sessions but returned when she elected to discontinue her acupuncture treatments – an economic decision.

FEEDBACK FROM FIRST SESSION:

Client slept throughout the last session. She says she felt totally relaxed and rejuvenated after the session. She went to bed earlier in the evening than normal and slept late the next day. There was no pain in her feet when she woke up.

FEEDBACK FROM SECOND SESSION:

Client says her feet were without pain most of the week. Her sleep cycles seem to have improved being awakened by hot flashes only twice during the night – she says otherwise 4 or 5 times was normal. Physical congestion in her feet is somewhat diminished.

FEEDBACK FROM THIRD SESSION:

Client says there has been no pain in her feet the entire week – only minimal at the end of the day and no throbbing at night. Hot flashes again seem improved with a frequency of 3 to 4 times per night on average.

FEEDBACK FROM FOURTH SESSION:

Client is extremely happy with the cessation of pain in her feet. The physical congestion is much less – almost indiscernible – remaining congestion is thinner and more fluid. Client reports that her sleep patterns continue to improve with an average of only about 3 hot flashes or less per night. Night sweats are diminished.

FEEDBACK FROM FIFTH SESSION:

There is virtually no physical congestion noted in the client s feet. This is a dramatic improvement with a client that I have been working with for over 50 foot reflexology sessions. Client reports that she is experiencing only 1 to 2 hot flashes at night and has, on occasion, experienced none at all throughout the night. She comes for sessions usually on a weekly schedule but, due to the holidays, it has been three weeks – still she is experiencing little or no pain in her feet. She says that her sleep had been disturbed in the past by her hot flashes, night sweats and the throbbing in her feet. She reports that those conditions have been corrected at this time. She says she has more energy and her mood has improved.

Patient's Age : 54 year Female

Diseases: Neck/Shoulders sensitivity Digestive discomfort Low back pain

Therapist : David Henry, NC USA

Result: SYMPTOMS:

Sensitivity in neck and shoulders lower back pain.

Occasional digestive discomfort with certain food types (particularly fatty foods).

NOTES:

Client reports gall bladder has been surgically removed as well as about 50 per cent of her thyroid in the early 90's. She suffers from low back pain at times and stiffness in her neck and shoulders (she indicates with her hand an area of the distal Levator scapularis and Spenius capitus).

Client is active, belongs to a gym where she swims 3 times weekly and does daily exercises. She is in training for a 60 mile walk for the Susan G Komen Breast Cancer Foundation. Currently, she is walking 15 miles per day. Her only medication is daily supplementation of vitamins/minerals. She says her life is comfortable – blames her cervical and lumbar sensitivity on long hours at her computer and her active lifestyle.

FEEDBACK FROM PATIENT AFTER 5TH SESSION:

I don't know exactly what the main difference is, except for the face work, but what ever you did this last time has made a huge difference!!! So much so that I want (if okay with you and your schedule) to continue what you are doing on a regular bi –weekly basis. You are on to something …the plan .... is a good one .....

so think which day is best for you on a bi–weekly time slot and let me know and then we'll get our ink pens out and make it a go.

Thank you.

Patient's Age : 26 years Male

Diseases: Cerebral paralysis

Therapist : Diane B, Canada

Result: I was able to do steps 1 and 2 during my first session.

From not being able to touch his face for more than 5 seconds, we are now able to do steps 1 and 2 completely!

I will keep you posted as to how things are going with my patient.

Patient's Age : 21 years Male

Diseases: Paralysis –Temporary caused by motor bicycle accident, right side of leg and foot especially

Therapist : Geri Karr, NC, USA

Result: I was asked to work with a 21 year old young boy, suffering a motor bicycle accident by his father. The boy is in rehabilitation and has been there approximately a month. He is getting his memory back in stages, has been walking, talking, writing, etc. However, he was in an accident back in November 2009 in which he was temporarily paralyzed on the right side, especially leg and foot. He is stuck in that period since mid-to end of week. He has lost use of his right leg and foot and says he is unable to feel anything. However, he did say when I began working with him that he could feel down to his knee.

During step 5 of facial reflexology, the boy began to move his right foot and toes when I was working the reflex area for the right leg and foot.

His father was so excited because his son could move his foot and toes that he went and got the head nurse to come in and watch him work that right foot after I finished the session. She was impressed and we briefly discussed your work.

Also, his father stated it is the first time since the accident that he has been still for 1 3/4 hours. He was very relaxed during the session and very excited about me coming back tomorrow afternoon. I got the best payment ever – a hug with a big smile and thank you.

Patient's Age : 62 year Male

Diseases: Stroke in the brain stem + stroke in the right occipital region

Therapist : Diane B, Canada

Result: I have done 6 facial reflex treatments with my brother who had a stroke in his brain stem and his right occipital region. I find his face looks much more alive after a session. He is very receptive to the treatment taking in deep breathes. For the first time he was able to undo his belt and button on his pants tonite!

Sometimes after a session he does a lot of good, common sense talking too! Long term and short term memory seems to be better. He also seems to be able to walk a bit better after a session. After the second session he said he felt like he had forgotten how to walk. I was a bit worried but once he stood up he was fine After the third session he said his brain seemed foggy for a short time.

After 4 sessions I was able to feel the plexus balancing pulse balance, the lymphatic points. The NP points are starting to balance as well as the crainial points. When I first started to work with him there were no pulses at all. He is taking quite a lot of medication right now.

Just letting you know that I have been doing the foot reflex therapy on my brother diligently 3 times per week.

This past week I noticed that the effects of the treatment were lasting for 2 days! This is very big in my eyes considering that they would not hold overnite before.

I have noticed that he is standing straighter, his face is balancing, he can get up off of my reflexology chair without any hesitation or help now, where as before, he needed help and it was a struggle for him.

I will continue to do the foot reflex therapy on him 3 times per week and see where it goes from here.

I am very very excited and happy for him! Very excited and happy that I can help him!

I am finding that the points on the right side are coming into balance more so than the ones on the left.

He still has a long way to go but we need to take one step at a time.

Thank you so much for putting together facial reflex therapy!

Patient's Age : 10 year old boy

Diseases: Genetic disorder (rare)

Therapist : Elisa Martinez Way, Denmark (Mother of John Patrick)

Result: JOHN PATRICK'S STORY

John Patrick is a happy 10 year old. He was born with a genetic disorder.

John Patrick's birth was long and problematic. After many hours of difficult labour it was necessary to deliver him by an emergency Caesarean-section. It was immediately apparent to the doctors who delivered him that something was wrong with him. The subsequent prolonged hospital stay was difficult for me and John Patrick.

To keep him alive, it was necessary to place John Patrick in an incubator. Unfortunately from the monitoring equipment, he received some terrible burns on his hands and feet.

After some time, we were told by the doctors that John Patrick had a rare genetic disorder. The only real prognosis we were told was that his life expectancy would be short. They told us that the genetic disorder which John Patrick had, amongst other things, would cause his inner organs to be deformed.

The doctors also informed us that his learning abilities would be impaired and their evaluation was not very encouraging. The prognosis of John Patrick living in a vegetative state for the rest of his life was a daunting prospect.

John Patrick was then subjected to a wide range of examinations which eliminated, amongst other things, the previously predicted deformity of his inner organs. The examinations also determined, more precisely, the nature of his condition.

From the beginning, things did not look good for John Patrick. He was a fragile child who needed a lot of care and attention. In the following years we were gradually able to see and define many of John Patrick s impairments.

We were unable to make eye-contact with him. We noticed when we picked him up from daycare he did not seem to recognize us and we later discovered that it was because his eyesight was really bad. John Patrick was unable to see us, because he had only 20 per cent visibility. His hearing was impaired and he had fluid in his ears. He lacked muscle tone, had problems with his balance and his feet were crooked. John Patrick had asthma and a lot of intestinal problems, amongst other problems.

I did everything that I possibly could to 'train' him. I was inspired by reading different books about learning and play techniques and massage for children. The main problem was that the majority of those books were designed for 'normal' children, but I persevered and massaged and trained John Patrick as well as I possibly could. I even got some positive results too.

Amongst other things, he learned to walk, keep his balance, eat by himself and play structurally. There were still a lot of other things that I didn t have the knowledge to help him with. A couple of those areas that I didn t know very much about were how to teach him social skills and fantasy play.

My main obstacle in training and helping John Patrick was the apparent lack of availability of qualified help or advice, so I was forced to search for the necessary tools and methods myself and try to apply them as best I could. Imagine my disappointment and frustration when it didn't work.

When John Patrick was 5 years old I met Lone Sorensen. I had been encouraged to take part in one of the courses she was running for parents of handicapped children. It was the first time that I had ever met a person who, not only understood what I was going through, but also knew and understood a lot about disabilities. I must admit that I was skeptical at first; I remember wondering, "Can so little stimulation really have such a big effect?"

I had, after all, struggled with massage, physical training, games and many other types of physically demanding activities. I was well aware of how much effort was needed just to achieve a little result. Here was a person who was telling me that by using only one and a half hours of stimulation a day, I would see obvious results after a very short time. At the same time, I just couldn't help but trust Lone – she gave me new hope, she made me feel that I was no longer alone in my efforts to stimulate and improve the life of my son.

Following the parent course I began to stimulate John Patrick with a type of pressure stimulation called Temprana therapy. John Patrick really enjoyed it and we both found that it was very pleasant for me to stimulate his face, hands and feet; we, very quickly built up a closer relationship.

After only a week of Temprana stimulation I began to see results. The process started with a cleansing of the body and as a result his asthma and intestinal problems became worse. He had an outbreak of asthma and eczema in many places on his body, but it didn't itch. This is apparently a normal reaction to the treatment.

During this period, I was constantly in touch with Lone who kept encouraging me to continue with the therapy.

I started seeing positive results within the first month – John Patrick stopped drooling and spitting up, it was such a great relief for me. John Patrick's balance became visibly better and he began to run around for the first time. I was able to hold prolonged eye contact with him; John Patrick started having eye contact with me throughout the entire stimulation session. The first time that happened tears ran down my cheeks – it was a wonderful feeling to suddenly have this connection with my son.

After 4 months of stimulation Temprana therapy, we went to see an orthopedic surgeon who remarked that his feet where less crooked – that for me was a major victory! John Patrick s asthma improved significantly and his intestinal problems were much better.

More and more positive and better results became apparent as the years went by. Some improvements happened quickly while others took longer.

Sometimes when one problem disappeared or showed improvement another previously present, but unknown one would appear and demand attention. This meant that Lone needed to constantly modify the treatment program to keep up with developments – this illustrates the high level of support and encouragement that I have received from Lone.

I have now been using Temprana therapy stimulation, a combination of facial, neuro foot and hand reflexology on John

Patrick for 5 years and the many positive results that we have achieved have vastly improved my son's quality of life.

Here is a list of the most remarkable ones:

His hearing has improved so much that he no longer needs a hearing aid.

He no longer suffers from asthma.

His intestinal problems are greatly improved.

His vision is now within normal parameters and he has good visual memory (it was only 20 per cent before!).

He plays computer games and has a high level of concentration.

His social abilities have improved from being virtually non-existent. Now he seeks play and contact with adults and other children.

He has a well developed sense of humor and likes to tease others (especially adults).

He has a strong self-will and is able to express it.

His general physical health has improved enormously.

He has shown great improvement in his personal abilities with everyday tasks such as; eating/drinking, dressing/undressing and helping with everyday tasks such as clearing up after himself.

I have no illusions about John Patrick s abilities. I am acutely aware that he will never be what is regarded as a 100 per cent normally functioning boy, but the improvement in his quality of life and his ability to function has definitely improved.

When I look at him today I see a boy who is living and exploring his life. Generally he has a happy and harmonic with nature, but sometimes does have a temper when he doesn't get his own way.

Lone Sorensen has given me an invaluable tool. Using Temprana therapy has made and will continue to make it possible to improve my son s ability to function well in a wide range of areas. Using Temprana therapy on John Patrick has also greatly improved my son s quality of life on a daily basis – a prospect that I never could have imagined when I first set out on this journey.

Patient's Age : 47 years Female

Diseases: Headaches (hormonal)

Therapist : Eva Duckert, Denmark

Result: For a long time the client had suffered from headaches and she is very surprised that just after 1 session with facial reflexology she almost never had headaches anymore. It is quite incredible.

Patient's Age : 57 years Female

Diseases: Headaches Sore neck, shoulder and arm

Therapist : Eva Duckert, Denmark

Result: Headaches and sore neck, shoulder and arm. For several years the client had headaches and sore neck, shoulder and arm, presumably from a fall. With 3 sessions of Tibetan neck treatment/ reflexology she has been free of her pain and she seldom needs painkillers, although they were a regular part of her morning ritual. (The client had been treated with physiotherapy for a year without any result and had also been treated by a chiropractor. Treatment helped for only a short time.)

Patient's Age : 57 years Female

Diseases: Headaches Neck and shoulder pain

Therapist : Eva Duckert, Denmark

Result: Since last week the client has had severe headache, neck and shoulder pain after she bumped her head into a door. When she left, there was still a little soreness in the neck and head but no pain. When she got home she called and told me that she had no soreness left and had full motion of the head/neck.

Patient's Age : 56 years Female

Diseases: Night blindness

Therapist : Eva Duckert, Denmark

Result: After just 4 treatments with ocular therapy/facial reflexology the client felt a perceptible shift in her eyes and she can now walk with her dogs when it is dark without feeling helpless.

Patient's Age : 52 years Female

Diseases: Severe stomach ache (from chemo tablets)

Therapist : Eva Duckert, Denmark

Result: Surgery two times and now on third chemotherapy because of ovarian cancer.

When she arrived, she did not mention (on purpose) that she had severe stomach pains. The chemo tablets, she gets, may cause volvulus, and is hard for the mucosa. I treated the patient with facial reflexology and I gave the client some points to treat at home to strengthen the immune system. And the next morning I got the sweetest email ... "Juhu - First morning without a stomach ache!"

Patient's Age : 24 years Female

Diseases: Sinusitis

Therapist : Eva Duckert, Denmark

Result: After a nasty sinus cold, the client developed problems with her sinuses. A session with facial reflexology caused the infection to come out the next day. The client was happy, when she could again breathe through her nose.

Patient's Age : 3 year old girl

Diseases: Cerebral Palsy + Microcephalia

Therapist : Gemza Senbursa, Turkey, Hacettepe University

Result: First results of research and systematic investigation to establish facts about Temprana reflex therapy done by a physiotherapist and student of Temprana reflex therapy, Gemza Senbursa in Turkey:

Four treatment groups:

1. Core stabilization exercises at home.

2. Core stabilization exercises + Manual therapy including mobilization and manipulation.

3. Core stabilization exercises + Kinesis-tape which is a special tape used in treatment – very popular all over the world

4. Core stabilization exercises + Facial reflex therapy.

I have three assessments – before treatment, after 8 sessions and one month later.

For every group, 20 patients were accepted.

I haven't finished statistics but all groups are progressing parallel to each other.

PATIENT REPORT:

Registrated change as follows:

Cerebral palsy + Microcephalia, 3 year old girl, after 17 sessions treatment:

a) She can open her eyes better.

b) Movements increased.

c) Stopped crying.

d) Eye contact is good and her gaze is more meaningful.

e) More peaceful.

f) Constipation finished.

g) Nutrition is better; she has put on weight.

Patient's Age : 9 year old girl

Diseases: Mental motor retardation

Therapist : Gemza Senbursa, Turkey, Hacettepe University

Result: First results of research and systematic investigation to establish facts about Temprana reflex therapy, done by

Physiotherapist and student of Temprana reflex therapy, Gemza Senbursa in Turkey :

Four treatment groups:

1.   Core stabilization exercises at home.

2.   Core stabilization exercises + Manual therapy including mobilization and manipulation

3.   Core stabilization exercises + Kinesis-tape which is a special tape used in treatment – very popular all over the world.

4.   Core stabilization exercises + Facial reflex therapy

I have three assessments – before treatment, after 8 sessions and one month later:-

For every group, 20 patients were accepted.

I haven't finished statistics but all the groups are progressing parallel to each other.

PATIENT REPORT:

Registrated change as follows:

Mental motor reterdation, 9 year old girl. After 15 session:

a.   She has started to say two word together like 'father come.'

b.   She use her mimics to convey things to others.

c.   More social.

d.   She can stay alone and watch television.

e.   Memory is better.

Patient's Age : 7 year old boy

Diseases: Mental motor reterdation + Autism

Therapist : Gemza Senbursa, Turkey, Hacettepe University

Result: First results of research and systematic investigation to establish facts about Temprana reflex therapy done by a physiotherapist and student of Temprana reflex therapy, Gemza Senbursa in Turkey:

Four treatment groups:

1. Core stabilization exercises at home.

2. Core stabilization exercises + Manual therapy including mobilization and manipulation

3. Core stabilization exercises + Kinesis-tape which is a special tape used in treatment – very popular all over the world.

4. Core stabilization exercise + Facial reflex therapy

I have three assessments – before treatment, after 8 sessions and one month later:-

For every group, 20 patients were accepted.

I haven't finished statistics but all the groups are progressing parallel to each other.

PATIENT REPORT:

Registrated change as follows:

Mental motor reterdation + Autism, 7 year old boy. After 10 sessions treatment:

a. He makes more sounds like, 'dede, baba, bambam.'

b. He is more interested in the environment.

c. Started to keep in touch with people, before he didn't.

d. More happy.

Patient's Age : 9 year old boy

Diseases: Mental motor reterdation + Autism

Therapist : Gemza Senbursa, Turkey, Hacettepe University

Result: First results of research and systematic investigation to establish facts about Temprana reflex therapy done by a Physiotherapist and student of Temprana reflex therapy, Gemza Senbursa in Turkey:

Four treatment groups:

1. Core stabilization exercises at home.

2. Core stabilization exercises + Manual therapy including mobilization and manipulation

3. Core stabilization exercises + Kinesis-tape which is a special tape used in treatment – very popular all over the world.

4. Core stabilization exercises + Facial reflex therapy

I have three assessments – before treatment, after 8 sessions and one month later:-

For every group, 20 patients were accepted.

I haven't finished statistics but all the groups are progressing parallel to each other.

PATIENT REPORT:

Registrated change as follows:

Mental motor reterdation + Autism, 9 year old boy. After 10 sessions treatment:

a. His gaze is more meaningful and investigates the environment.

b. Stopped smiling when it is meaningless.

c. Peevishness increased.

d. His responses got organised than before.

Patient's Age : 6 year old girl

Diseases: Mental motor reter-dation, Cerebral palsy Epilepsy

Therapist : Gemza Senbursa, Turkey, Hacettepe University

Result: First results of research and systematic investigation to establish facts about Temprana reflex therapy done by a Physiotherapist and student of Temprana reflex therapy, Gemza Senbursa in Turkey:

Four treatment groups:

1.   Core stabilization exercises at home.

2.   Core stabilization exercises + Manual therapy including mobilization and manipulation

3.   Core stabilization exercises + Kinesis-tape which is a special tape used in treatment – very popular all over the world.

4.   Core stabilization exercises + Facial reflex therapy

I have three assessments – before treatment, after 8 sessions and one month later:-

For every group, 20 patients were accepted.

I haven't finished statistics but all the groups are progressing parallel to each other.

PATIENT REPORT:

Registrated change as follows:

Mental motor reterdation, cerebral palsy and epilepsy, 6 year old girl. After 23 sessions:

a.   Spasticity is less.

b.   She can sit all day without support.

c.   Sleeps good.

d.   Try to grab things with hands.

e.   Extend her arms to touch her hair.

g.   Makes sounds.

h.   Concerned with the environment.

i.   Know her name.

j.   Looks the sounds are coming.

k.   Watches television.

l.   She had a deviation in her which eyes now looks more normal.

Patient's Age : 30 years Female

Diseases: Headaches

Therapist : Hanne Bundgaard, Denmark

Result: She suffered from headaches, which she has had daily since last 8-9 months.

After 8 sessions of facial reflexology, the headaches have disappeared and she has not had any pain in the last 5-6 weeks.

Patient's Age : 45 years Male

Diseases: Trigeminal neuralgia Post-viral fatigue

Therapist : Helen Wood, Bingley, West Yorkshire, UK

Result: My client is a 45 years old male who was suffering from trigeminal neuralgia and post-viral fatigue. These symptoms occurred shortly after contracting a cold virus, in March 2009 and have not eased since. Until contracting this virus, he had always been a very physically active man. He would cycle a 30 mile round trip to work and back home every day, attend a martial arts group 3 evenings a week, and was always motivated to turn his hand to any activity he was interested in. Since his illness, he had been barely able to attend his martial arts group at all. Initially he was off work for a month, as his energy levels were reduced to zero. He described the pains in the right side of his face and throat as excruciating, and his general physician arranged various scans and blood tests for him. However, they were all inconclusive. The only diagnosis that could be made was that of a virus, and it was told it was just a matter of rest and time until the symptoms pass. He was prescribed painkillers and asked to be patient by his specialist.

FEEDBACK AFTER FIFTH TREATMENT

He hasn't had any flare up of his physical symptoms, and feels so much better. His fatigue has completely gone, and he can exercise daily without any unpleasant symptoms of fatigue. He still has a slight tenderness on his jaw and his doctor has reduced his medication further. His doctor has expressed his interest in rapid recovery, and the facial reflexology sorensensistemTM treatment! He has never before seen symptoms of trigeminal neuralgia reduced so rapidly in one of his patients.

I will aim to gradually increase the time between appointments from weekly to fortnightly, and eventually from three weekly to monthly provided there is an absence of symptoms, until a full recovery has been made.

Patient's Age : 9 year old twin boys

Diseases: Cerebral palsy

Therapist : Lone Sorensen, Denmark Helle, Denmark (written by mother of Johan and Jesper)

Result: A MOTHER'S STORY

I'll just have to write to you, because I am so filled with joy today. My greatest sorrow in connection with the boys' disability was that I could not be alone with them and always have a helper in the house when Jørgen is not at home.

Today I had the boys alone. Jesper came home at 1 p.m. and I did Temprana therapy with him. Then we picked up Johan at his school, came home and the boys were playing together (yes you read right) and then Jesper was playing with water at the sink while I did Temprana with Johan. I cooked dinner together with Jesper, while Johan played the television games.

We had dinner together and had a lovely time.

Jesper had a shower, while Johan again played the television games and I was ready to put both children to bed when Jørgen came home.

It has been a most pleasant and enjoyable day.

The best thing is that the boys have started playing together and now Jesper also wants to play with Johan. So much progress has happened with both boys, but perhaps most visibly with Jesper, who must know everything that happens around him.

Jesper goes so well when I support him under his arms. Now he runs away bearing his own weight. So even though he has been to the toilet 3 times and in / out of the car seat I have no back pain today.

Both the physiotherapist, (to help us with options of Jesper's aids) and the consultant (who creates the new indoor electric wheelchair to Jesper) can see the changes:-

The physiotherapist has said that if Jesper is going to walk, then we have his full attention.... The physiotherapist is also working at Hvidovre Hospital and collaborates with the boys' pediatrician Søren Anker, a highly regarded pediatrician in Denmark and MR. BOTOX himself. So it will definitely be interesting to get that way around ...

Johan still has many 'outages' and 'attacked' Jesper again last Sunday by scratching him very much in the face when we were at our farmhouse and just had to struggle with something in the bus while the boys were inside the house. But his play has evolved a lot and he may be free of my attention, sometimes, like today.

So I would basically just tell you I am so grateful that you have spent so much time of your life developing Temprana .... I can not describe it with words – for they are not enough ... but I feel we have a GREAT chance given away to improve the boys and our lives.

Patient's Age : 23 years Female

Diseases: Thyroid gland Headaches Heart problems Sleeping-problems

Therapist : Ilona Sobelewska Poland

Result: Symptoms:

1. Thyroid gland condition.

2. Headaches

3. Heart problems.

4. Problems with sleeping.

5. Bad hair and nail condition.

6. Back pain.

7. Becoming overly anxious and stressed.

AFTER 8 SESSIONS

Patient much calmer and happier, more energetic, still eating a lot!! Falls asleep during the sessions much quicker now. Some of the nerve points found particularly painful.

Another 2 sessions are to be carried out tomorrow and the day after tomorrow, followed by nerve point stimulation, 3 times a week for another month.

This, however, will be done by the patient's partner as they both live in Liverpool and I am staying here only till Sunday.

SUMMARY

Patient feels much calmer and relaxed during the treatment period. Has had a good night sleep. Not a single headache!!! Nor back pain.

Much more energetic and less anxious. As for the improvement of the thyroid gland activity, the patient will be doing some blood tests next month to check any changes.

Patient's Age : 58 year Male

Diseases: Parkinson's disease

Therapist : Jo Ann, NC, USA

Result: Former parachute jumping soldier who broke every bone in his body it seems.

Major complaint: Parkinson's disease for nine years.

Medications: On lots of medicines.

SYMPTOMS:

Stiff muscles all over the body. Tremors are under control due to medications.

Sharp stabbing pain in feet upon rising. These pains are short and then go away. He gave pain color = green. Arms and first three fingers of each arm go numb 10-12 times a day. Very bad and unrelenting. He gives the pain color = red. I feel the arm, numbness and pain in fingers is due to the seventh cervical vertebra being out of line. Client does not go to a chiropractor but has been encouraged to do so.

THIRD SESSION:

Client reports that after about one hour he experienced more pain and discomfort following our last session. Then he had a period of 8 hours of relief from pain so he could actually fall asleep in his reclining chair and slept all night till 6:00 a.m. The first real night s sleep in a long time.

FORTH SESSION:

Client is pleased with the relief from pain he is experiencing although pain does return.

FIFTH SESSION:

Client happy with results and says he feels better after his sessions.

Patient's Age : 28 month old boy

Diseases: Verbal ability, Lack of

Therapist : Jo Ann, NC, USA

Result: 28 month old boy is not talking yet. Although he has a speech therapist, his mother feels she would like to try facial reflexology in addition to his other therapy. He seems to understand well and can non-verbally communicate his wishes quite well with grunts and pointing.

FIFTH SESSION:

Our little boy is now saying three word sentences on a regular basis. Mother is very pleased.

Treatment was the same as the second session but only to the extent he would tolerate. He doesn't mind cranial lines and points while his mother reads or plays with him. He is more comfortable with me and doesn't seem to mind our sessions as much.

I recommend we continue once a week if it is possible.

Patient's Age : 6 $^1/_2$ year old

Diseases: Dyspraxia Oral and verbal Temprana therapy

Therapist : Joan Vendelboe Nielsen, Denmark

Result: Lucas was my first temprana reflex therapy child. He was also my examination case.

Lucas is a bright, happy and co-operative boy. His biggest wish was to be understood. It has been difficult for him because Lucas had oral and verbal dyspraxia.

At 6 $^1/_2$ years, Lucas verbal language ability was graded to only 50 per cent in fluency. This means his verbal communication only consisted of monosyllable words like house, mom, dad, car, etc. After 2-3 months of Temprana reflex therapy there was a considerable change in Lucas. This was seen physically, psychologically and verbally. He began to pronunce more sounds and more words.

After 4-6 months of Temprana reflex therapy he could pronounce polysyllable words and construct simple sentences. His pronounication improved and his verbal language results were graded to 25 per cent in fluency.

The following months he progressed profusely. Lucas was now able to complete sentences and his articulation improved. After about one year of Temprana reflex thearpy, Lucas s verbal communication skills are graded to 100 per cent in fluency. This of course has had a positive effect on Lucas s social life, as now he is understood. Most of all, it has boosted his self-esteem and he is no longer afraid to interact with others and no longer feels socially isolated.Temprana reflex therapy is the most unique and effective treatment I have ever known. I am so grateful that I have had the opportunity to study this therapy form.

Patient's Age : 5 year old boy

Diseases: Autism

Therapist : Lone Sorensen, Denmark

Result: MEDICAL DIAGNOSIS IN 2004: AUTISM

Prognosis: Extremely slow learning abilities. No prospect for normal learning or schooling. No prospect for an independent life.

OBSERVATIONS: FEBRUARY 2005

Low verbal ability – can only compile a maximum of 2 words.

Low verbal understanding (that is, hot - cold, happy - sad).

Inability for self-expression.

Good eye contact, but is absent for shorter moments, several times during the day.

Very aggressive behavior – bad temper is shown by throwing himself on the floor and crying.

Doesn't have repetitive tendencies (this behavior pattern was shown when he was younger).

Good contact with other children and adults.

GROSS MOTOR SKILLS:

Good gross motor skills fine, but has problems keeping his balance.

Potty trained.

Does not have the ability to bike.

Does not have the ability to swim.

FINE MOTOR SKILLS:

Eats and drinks by himself.

Scribbles, but uses only one color.

PRIMARY DIET :

Milk.

Refined white flour.

Sugar.

Processed food heated in the microwave.

DIETARY SUPPLEMENTS:

None.

Tristan lives alone with his mother Ulla. Tristan s grandmother lives in the same building and he visits her frequently. His parents are divorced and they have a dysfunctional relationship. Ulla explains she had many problems with her relationship with the father during and after the pregnancy. Ulla believes that Tristan's condition is a result of this situation. The parents still have a dysfunctional relationship and they are going through a court case. Tristan visits his father every third weekend and during the summer vacation. Tristan goes to a kindergarten for children with special needs. MEDICAL DIAGNOSIS 2005: AUTISTIC TRAITS. Prognosis: Slow learning abilities. Prospect for learning in a special needs school. Prospect of no independent life.

Observations and changes compared to the last consultation: February 2006: Normal verbal ability, but does have some pronunciation problems.

Perfect verbal understanding (that is, hot – cold, happy – sad).

Ability to express himself.

Good eye contact.

Does not loose his temper as often and is not aggressive anymore.

Does not have repetitive tendencies.

Good contact with other children and adults.

Loves to play with other children and loves to walk to the kindergarten.

GROSS MOTOR SKILLS:

No balance problems.

Potty trained.

Is able to bike.

Is able to swim.

Is able to dance.

FINE MOTOR SKILLS:

Eats and drinks by himself.

Draws figures, people, houses, trees, etc.

DIET:

Does not drink milk.

Eats refined flour.

Eats sugar once in a while.

Eats a wholesome and well balanced diet.

DIET SUPPLEMENT:

Omega 3

Tristan would like to learn to play the violin.

JANUARY 2007

Tristan has started going to a normal school.

Patient's Age : 18 year old girl

Diseases: Anorexia Lack of menstruation

Therapist : Joanna Wilder, Danmark

Result: In November last year I had a young 18 year old skinny little client who had symptoms of anorexia.

She came to me because she had abdominal pain, and because she had not menstruated for a year.

After 2 sessions she started menstruating again, and I've heard it continues on a regular basis yet.

She was very fond of my sessions, quite apart from the deep relaxing effect. She felt it was a miracle with her menstuation and after 4 sessions I could feel she was more happy, open and positive. One day she came in confused regarding a decision; very confused in her head, but after the session, she was fully aware of her head and had found the answer to her problem. She would like to discuss her somewhat fanatical eating habits with me (she did not use the word anorexia herself). She told me, she had emotional baggage that might be the cause of her situation.

I think that she came to an understanding of herself and found a context of her situation.

She knew the abdominal pain most likely was emotional tensions and hunger – to put it bluntly.

What I want to say at last is that the treatment seemed very positive for the mental part of this case.

Patient's Age : 56 years Female

Diseases: Arthritis pain, stiff / sore lower back, Insomnia

Therapist : Josefine Lebeck Hentze, Denmark

Result: Treatment with facial reflexology and neuro-foot reflexology.

3 sessions at 1 week intervals, 1 session, 6 weeks after the third session.

Conclusion: Low back stiffness and soreness kept getting better and better with each session. The good effect had stuck to the fourth session, however, she felt a slight deterioration, the more time that passed from the third session. After the fourth session, her lower back improved further and she commented that she could stoop better while gardening than she had for many years. Furthermore, there had been a favorable effect on her edema which had diminished since sessions had started.

She had less arthritic pain in the wrist and ankle; she could go for longer walks without pain.

She experienced that she was clearer in her head after the sessions.

After 4 sessions she also had less pain in the hip.

I treated her insomnia in the fourth session and it helped her immediately. I gave her some facial reflexology points to treat at home every night or if she woke up at night and could not fall asleep again. It did really well. She had been given sleeping pills for many years but had stopped taking them not so long ago. Facial reflexology is a good alternative to sleeping pills – and without side effects.

The client had previously tried many other therapies including acupuncture, but it was only with facial reflexology, she experienced that an alternative form of treatment really worked on her.

Patient's Age : 58 years Female

Diseases: Back problems and arthritis

Therapist : Josefine Lebeck Hentze, Denmark

Result: Last summer I had a client whom I treated once a week for about 4 sessions in total, and each time she came, her back was better and she could go better and be active without arthritic pain.

Patient's Age : 69 years Male

Diseases: Cataract with distance focus problem

Therapist : Lila, USA

Result: FACIAL REFLEXOLOGY, SPECIAL EYE TREATMENT:

Facial reflexology with eye reflex therapy was performed. Following the treatment, he indicated that he could focus better and items seemed closer to him.

Patient's Age : 59 years Male

Diseases: Dry eye, extreme

Therapist : Lila, USA

Result: FACIAL REFLEXOLOGY, SPECIAL EYE TREATMENT:

Facial reflexology with eye reflex therapy was performed. During the eye treatment, tears flowed into his eyes.

Patient's Age : 88 years Female

Diseases: Macular degeneration

Therapist : Lila, USA

Result: FACIAL REFLEXOLOGY, SPECIAL EYE TREATMENT:

After one facial reflexology with eye reflex therapy treatment, she was able to see shadows. She had not been able to see anything for years.

Facial Reflexoloy Schools in the World

Main Institute: International Institute of Facial and Temprana Reflex Therapy, Barcelona, Spain:

sorensensistem@post.tele.dk   www.reflexologiafacial.es

Australian

reflexologyaustralia@gmail.com

www.reflexologyaustralia.com

Argentina

centrodereflexologia@arnet.com.ar

www.reflexologiafacial.es

Rosario- Santa Fe

monilopez@yahoo.com

Checz Republic

miro@miro-cz.eu

www.miro-cz.eu

Dubai and Abu Dhabi

julieg@eim.ae

www.juliegreenhalgh.com

Denmark

ddz@ddz.dk

www.ddz-herlev.dk

England

nikke.ariff@btinternet.com

www.facialreflexology.com

penny@libra-reflexology.co.uk

www.libra-reflexology.co.uk

Finland   info@nictab.se

www.nictab.se

Greece

robert.przybys@gmail.com

www.temprana.pl/gr/

Holland

gezichtsreflexologie@hotmail.com

www.reflex-zonetherapie.nl

México

centrobodhisattva@hotmail.com

Veracruz, Mexico

olarayial@yahoo.com.mx

Japan

ayako@imsi.co.jp

www.imsi.co.jp

Poland

beasek@go2.pl

www.refleksoterapia.net.pl

robert.przybys@gmail.com

www.temprana.pl

majakrauze@op.pl   www.majakrauze.pl

USA

tswyat@bellsouth.net

www.reflexology-nc.org

Sweden, Norway

anna@kropphalsa.se

www.kropphalsa.se

irene@beroringspunkten.se

www.beroringspunkten.se

rosita@facepower.se

www.facepower.se

Spain, Madrid

info@divertilates.es

www.divertilates.es

Bibliography

Enciclopedia de Medicina
Dr Alfredo Embid
Association of Complementary Medicine
Published by AMC 1998
Madrid, Spain

La Nasal Terapia
Ludmilda de Bardo
Published by Mandala 1992
Madrid, Spain

Manual de Acupuntura
Dr. Orlando A Rigor
Published by Ecimed & Published by Science Doctor
Havana, Cuba

Diagnostico clinico
Jose Leon-Carrion
Published by Alfar, 1986
Seville, Spain

Bases Neurobiologicas de las Reflexoterapias
Dr Juan Bossy
Published by Masson S.A. 1999
Paris, France

Cibertherapy
Dr Caballo, Cuba 1990

Introduktion i Klassisk Akupunktur
Per Lauborg
Published by Forlaget Sopela 1984
Denmark

La Medicina Rescartada
Dr. Jose Campos & Dr. Geraldo Domingos Coelho
Published by Errepar,1984
Argentina

Educational material from the Institute of Facial & Foot
Reflexology
Lone Sorensen
sorensensistem, 1980-2003

Resources

INTERNATIONAL INSTITUTE OF FACIAL AND FOOT REFLEXOLOGY

Lone Sorensen

Lope de Vega 6, 08005 Barcelona, Spain
(0034) 932655700

Sorensensistem@post.tele.dk
www.reflexologiafacial.es
www.lonesorensen.com
www.temprana.org

About the Author

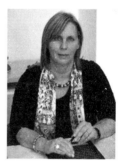

Lone Sorensen had her professional education from 1978 until 1985 in Reflexology, Acupuncture and Laser Therapy in Denmark. Lone always had a great interest in helping children, so she went to Germany to study cranial therapy work. By that time Lone had 19 diplomas in various worldwide additional therapy courses mostly studied in German and English, but she was always wanting more information about therapies she could work with about children's problems and this gave her great experience in the diagnosis of many children's illnesses. She developed Facial Reflexology during 26 years of research and intensive work in Denmark and South America. She took Reflexology to Argentina and founded the first three schools in that country. She also studied in Chile, Cuba, France, Spain and Germany. She has taken part in many conventions, national as well as international. In march 2001, Lone Sorensen was awarded by the **O.M.H.S.** with three Nobility prizes, becoming this way in the first reflexologist in the world to obtain such a mention, for her work in Zone therapy, Foot and Hand Reflexology and Facial Reflexology.

Reflexology
A way to better health

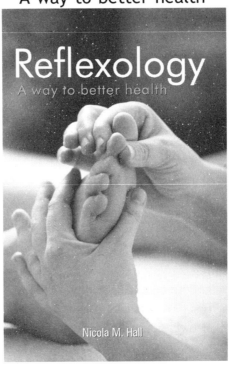

- Illustrative diagrams with the proper labeling
- Symptoms of 100 common disorders along with the type and way of reflexology needed given
- A detailed discussion on anatomical zones and its importance in reflexology
- Clinical cases to aid in better understanding

ISBN No.: 978-81-319-0508-1 | Pages: 188 | Price: ₹ 99.00

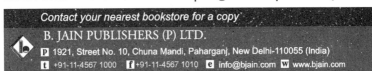

Contact your nearest bookstore for a copy

B. JAIN PUBLISHERS (P) LTD.

P 1921, Street No. 10, Chuna Mandi, Paharganj, New Delhi-110055 (India)
t +91-11-4567 1000 f +91-11-4567 1010 e info@bjain.com w www.bjain.com